COMA, A HEALING JOURNEY

AMY MINDELL, PH.D.

COMA, A HEALING JOURNEY

A GUIDE FOR
FAMILY,
FRIENDS
AND HELPERS

INTRODUCTION BY ARNOLD MINDELL

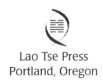

Lao Tse Press
Portland, Oregon

Distributed to the trade by Words Distributing Company, 7900 Edgewater Drive, Oakland, CA 94621.

Printed in the United States of America

Book design by Kate Jobe
Illustrations by Robert King

Mindell, Amy
    Coma, A Healing Journey: a guide for family, friends and helpers
    Bibliography
    Includes index.
ISBN 1-887078-05-3 (pbk.)
Library of Congress Catalog Card Number: 98-88184

Contents

List of Illustrations

Acknowledgments

This book would not be possible if it weren't for the pioneering work of Arnold Mindell, my partner and husband. His process-oriented coma work has been a healing balm for so many comatose adults and children and their families, who have been in desperate need. Arny's work brings a soothing light to some of the most painful and lonely corners of life. This manual is a product of his discoveries and research, and our collaborative experiences and learnings.

Many thanks to Nisha Zenoff, who contributed to this book so personally by discussing the intimate details of how she assisted her mother through her comatose state just before death. Nisha's gift of communicating her experiences helps make coma work more tangible and accessible.

My thanks to Ursi Jean and Dr. Pierre Morin in Switzerland, whose own work with comatose patients and their feedback about this manual have been invaluable to me. I am especially grateful to Gerri Haynes, whose work with hospice and with the dying, as well as her immense heart and helpful feedback, have been tremendous sources of inspiration and knowledge for me. Many thanks to Kay Ross for her ability to connect medical and nursing methods to coma work and her teaching of both worlds, and to Stan Tomandl for his constant support in this work, for always providing literature resources, and for his ability over the years to formulate and make accessible coma work concepts. Thanks also to Renata Ackermann and Kate Jobe for their feedback about this work and to Gary Reiss for his generosity in sharing learning about his work with comatose patients and their families. I am very appreciative of Dr. Ela Biede and Dr. Ernie Stewart for their medical knowledge of comatose states and the bridges of connection they provided to process-oriented thinking.

Thanks to Jane Kepner for her very helpful research skills and to Tom Osborne for his literature support. Margaret Ryan was a most skilled and loving editor of the work, who brought humor and compassion in the midst of editing. Sandra Dorr's clear advice and editing were crucial in the early stages of writing. Many thanks to Mary McAuley for her detailed and loving editing in the manuscript's last stages. Thanks also to Sonja Straub, Lane Arye, Herb Long, Ingrid and Stephen Schuitevoerder, Salome Schwarz, Dawn

Menken, Renata Ackermann, Kate Jobe, Lily Vassiliou, and Helena Lee for their individual contributions I am very appreciative of Debbie Hart, Kay Ross, Emetchi, Lily Vassiliou, and Richard Grimaldi for helping create the original photographs for this manual. I also want to mention Dimi Reber, my dance teacher at Antioch College, whose teaching helped illuminate the beauty and wisdom of movement.

I am especially grateful to Robert King for his beautiful illustrations. Robert has the uncanny capacity to transform photographs into living, breathing drawings that illuminate with simplicity and grace the essence of coma work. His artistic ability highlights special qualities of coma work and makes it possible for the reader to grasp coma methods in an immediate and deeply-felt way.

I am also strongly indebted to those courageous pioneers who have braved the mostly forbidden worlds of near-death experiences, dying, and comatose states: Elizabeth Kubler-Ross, Ondrea and Stephen Levine, Raymond Moody, Kenneth Ring, and many others.

Many thanks to all of our seminar participants around the world and my class participants at the Process Work Center of Portland, who have experimented with and tested the teaching concepts and exercises in this book. Their friendship and feedback have been invaluable to me.

Mostly, I want to thank all of those individuals in comatose states with whom we have worked, as well as their families and friends. We have shared many deep moments together, and I am eternally grateful for so much that I have learned from all of you about life, death, and the many mysteries we human beings encounter.

Coma, *A Healing Journey* is the most comprehensive and detailed description of nonviolent coma work that exists today. Until now, approaches to coma that we know of, including medical and nonmedical treatments, have emphasized shocking, pinching, and other kinds of aggressive or noxious stimulation based on the pathological model; the person in a comatose state must adapt and return immediately to everyday reality.

While process work does not deny the potential usefulness of such approaches, they seem unnecessarily violent. Instead, coma work is based on the philosophy that the human being in a coma is on an inner journey, dealing with that coma in the best way nature knows how. Therefore our entire effort is devoted to meeting individuals where they are, in that deepest, almost unfathomable, altered state of consciousness. In other words, instead of arresting the coma state, we encourage and join the comatose person in exploring that journey. In this way, the comatose person has a chance of feeling related to. Empathy with that state results in a heightened communication potential and, occasionally, awesome insights and contact. That's our goal: to assist the person in a coma either to direct or, at least, to take part in her or his healing program.

If we remember that, in the words of medical experts, today's medical treatment for coma is still in the dark ages and bound to improve in the near future, the kind of explicit, detailed, and compassionate communication Amy's book leads us through will stand independent of time. Regardless of medical progress, *Coma, A Healing Journey* will remain a central means of dealing with both the pathological state of coma and its potential purposefulness. Her method will always be applicable, regardless of the century we're living in.

Arnold Mindell

For your safety and mine: *nothing* in this book is intended for use without medical supervision.

I began writing this book when I suddenly realized that there are thousands of family members and friends of people in comas who feel desperate, alone, and abandoned in the face of the deepest of all unconscious states. The coma condition is starkly different from the rest of life's states of being. If the human being is in pain and dealing with a normal state of consciousness, just about anybody can find something to do to help that person. The torment of experiencing the disappearance of a loved one into a comatose state is an unparalleled agony. The concerned relative or friend is then further distressed by the blank expressions on the well-meaning faces of medical helpers, expressions indicating that a person in a coma is no longer "really" present.

Coma, A Healing Journey addresses this agony by providing relatives and caregivers with practical and sensitive methods of communicating directly with loved ones in coma. Part I provides a general introduction to and theoretical knowledge about coma work. Parts II and III consist of two manuals.

Part II is geared toward family members and friends who are in crisis because a loved one has fallen into a coma. If you are such a family member, you can turn immediately to Part II for helpful methods of communicating with your loved one. Put this book by his or her bedside, and use it as a step-by-step guide.

Part III is geared toward professional helpers, therapists, nurses, doctors, and hospice personnel who interact with comatose individuals and their families. Part III guides you and your colleagues through a progressive, in-depth training in coma work. The methods can be practiced with a few of your colleagues or in a classroom situation.

Again, for your safety and mine, I must add: *nothing* in this book is intended for use without medical supervision.

This book came about as a result of a number of factors. First, it was inspired by the many dramatic and extraordinary experiences that have emerged through the kinds of communication taught in this book. Together, my husband and partner, Arny, and I and colleagues have worked with people using these techniques (which grew out of Arny's work with comatose people) in many parts of the world. As a result, I felt pressed from deep within myself to offer not just the theory but a training process for anyone who needs to communicate with a person in a comatose state. My hope is that *Coma: A Healing Journey* will provide assistance and sustenance to many people just as our individual work has helped those whom we could reach within our physical boundaries.

Second, this manual came about because of the realization that practically all of us will be touched by coma in some way during our lives, yet we are unprepared as to how to deal with this altered state of consciousness. Many of us know someone who has fallen suddenly into a coma as a result of a brain injury—perhaps a child, a teenager, or an adult. Others have been at the bedside of a relative or a friend who has lapsed into a coma before death. Most of us know someone who has fallen into a coma as a result of illnesses such as cancer or acquired immunodeficiency syndrome (AIDS). Many of us have experienced a coma of varying duration during some part of our lives, and most people will enter into a comatose state just near death.

Third, this book is also a response to the questions we are asked repeatedly about coma work and how to use these skills with family members and friends in comatose states. The vast majority of calls we receive for coma assistance pertain to comas resulting from brain injury. This has surprised us because Arny's book (*Coma*, published in 1989) focused mainly on work with people in comas resulting

from near-death conditions. Yet, many of the situations we have encountered have involved people of varying ages who are in comas attributable to near-drowning, traumatic injuries such as violent blows to the head, bicycle accidents, strokes, car accidents, and suicide attempts. I recognized the need for the explication of tools for working with all types of coma, particularly those comas resulting from brain injury. In *Coma, A Healing Journey* I describe in detail the coma methods we have developed for working with people in all types of coma, including in near-death conditions, and special methods for working with brain-injured individuals.

Fourth, this manual grew out of the realization that a longer and more intensive coma training was needed so that students could delve intensively into learning the skills and methods of coma work. Over the last six years I have developed this course in Portland, Oregon, and, in the last year, with the help of Kay Ross, RN. The tools in this book are helpful, and to this date coma work has had only beneficial effects. Nonetheless, there is no substitute for live, hands-on training when possible.

I also realized that, while the methods in this book are geared toward communicating with people in comatose states, they are more widely applicable. The methods are helpful in communicating with people in withdrawn, internal states or assisting people who are ill. The inner work, movement, and body work methods in this book are generally helpful for anyone who wants to explore and value her or his deep inner processes.

It did not really surprise me that I was drawn strongly to working with people in comatose states. I seem to have been preconditioned from childhood. Much of my childhood days I spent whirling around trees singing songs, dancing and expressing the inexpressible. Whenever possible, I locked myself in my room in order to spend precious time painting, playing my guitar, and singing.

From the age of five through my days at Antioch College, I studied many forms of dance—including ballet, tap, jazz, modern, African—and improvisation, choreography, and many other movement forms including mime, clowning, and t'ai chi ch'uan. My studies of dance history, dance therapy, and shamanism expanded my knowledge of the healing quality of movement, the use of ritual dances from around the world as a means to get closer to God, and the interface between movement and many forms of body work.

Through immersing myself in body and movement training for so many years, I came to realize how important these frequently less appreciated modes of communication can be in interacting with people in special circumstances. My work at a state-run retardation center and a recreational department in a children's hospital, as well as my studies of dance therapy, further impressed upon me the necessity of altering one's communication style, particularly with people who do not communicate in traditional verbal ways. I was pressed to develop the use of sound, movement, gesture, hands-on contact, and artwork to get close to many individuals. I realized that it is up to the caregiver or therapist, not the client, to make this effort to bridge the gap that arises when "normal" communication channels are unavailable.

My ensuing interest in psychology spurred me toward becoming a therapist. I searched for a therapeutic modality in which I would be free to vary my style depending on the nature of my client. In 1981 I went to Zurich to study process-oriented psychology, which we call process work for short. I discovered a therapeutic form in which movement, art, and verbal therapy were intricately interwoven. A central tenet of process work is that any symptom is potentially meaningful, that there are worlds to discover in the often painful and seemingly meaningless areas of life. People are not only sick but full of potential.

I have always been an altered-state kind of person—dreamy, thoughtful, staring at the birds, and full of fantasy. I have often felt like a misfit, unable to adapt to ordinary reality, longing to bring my flights of fantasy into my life as a whole. Perhaps that is why I feel at home with people in comas. I was delighted to find that there is actually a science behind altered states—a science that connects to coma, the deepest altered state of all.

Amy Mindell,
Portland, Oregon

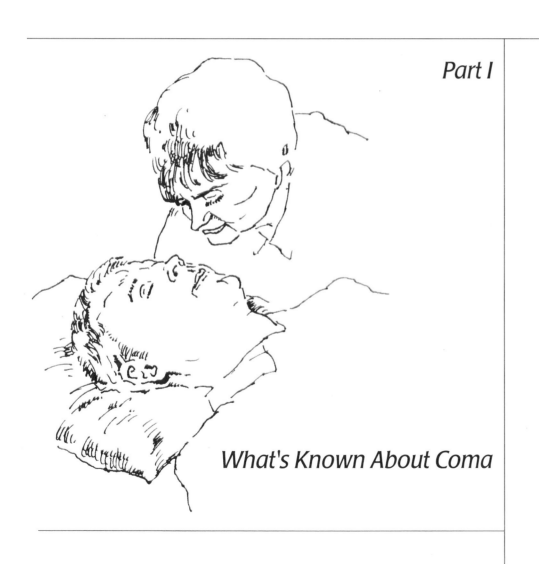

Part I

What's Known About Coma

W hen I arrived home late last night and listened to the answering machine, I was not really surprised by the woman's tone of urgency and desperation. Such calls have become common in our home. She wanted help in communicating with her mother, who had fallen into a coma as a result of a car accident. I didn't know this woman at all, but her plight had become all too familiar to me.

Coma is always shocking. Although the best medical procedures efficiently attend to the immediate needs and vital care of the body of the person, we are left with a traumatic and unavoidable gap between ourselves and the comatose person. It is estimated that in the United States there are 4000 to 10,000 children and 10,000 to 25,000 adults in long-term coma (or persistent vegetative state).[1] In Switzerland, where we lived previously, the statistics are just slightly lower.[2] Other studies suggest that there are approximately 500,000 new cases of head injury (one of the leading causes of coma) per year in the United States[3], and that twenty-five percent of these are categorized as leading to a persistent vegetative state.[4] Coma affects people from all walks of life—from little children to elderly individuals—and from all cultures.

This training guide creates a bridge between relatives and caretakers and the inner journey of a comatose person. It includes special communication methods for assisting individuals in a comatose state to follow their inner experiences. This method assumes that the person is not simply lost to coma, but is going through potentially meaningful inner experiences, and that, after all possible medical emergencies and causes are cared for, we can communicate with the person through special methods.

The methods help relieve some of the frustration and loneliness of feeling so out of contact with the comatose person. They also make it possible to connect lovingly with the comatose person and enable that person to communicate with us. This book is about accompanying people through the nighttime journey of coma by the light of the moon, that is, by their own nighttime consciousness.

> **Note: This is two books in one, if you (or someone near you) have a loved one in a coma and need immediate access to tools for working with that person,** you can jump directly to Part II. Put this book by the bedside of your loved one, and use it as a step-by-step guide.
>
> **Note: If you are a caretaker interested in in-depth instruction,** you and your colleagues will find, first, theoretical information in Part I. Then you can skip to Part III, where you will find a progressive, in-depth training guide.

The Story of Peter

In 1986 Arny and I were vacationing in the Swiss mountains. A woman named Sandy, now a good friend of ours, phoned. Her thirty-eight-year-old husband had acute leukemia and was not expected to live long. Sandy begged Arny to come to the city and work with him in the hospital. She felt that Arny's therapeutic work with body symptoms would be of help to her husband.

Arny and I were just beginning our relationship, and he asked me to go with him and participate in the work with Peter's wife and family. I didn't know at that time that the experiences we would share with this man would change my life—and would also be the beginning of this book.

We worked with Peter and his family for months. His leukemia was progressing rapidly, and he was told that he did not have long to live. I noticed that Peter, though cordial and kind, was quite shy with me whenever I saw him. One day, I was on my way to teach a class on movement and psychology in downtown Zurich and decided to stop in briefly to say hello to Peter. When I arrived at the hospital, the doctor told me that I could not go in the room. He said that Peter had fallen into a coma and was going to die that night. Only Sandy was allowed in the room.

I telephoned Arny and told him to come to the hospital. I also made contact with Sandy, who insisted that we be allowed in the room. I raced to my class in an utter frenzy to tell them that I would not be able to teach that evening.

When we entered Peter's room, I was shocked. I had never been with anyone who was dying. My whole body quaked. Peter looked so different from the man I had known before. He was lying down, his skin was pale, his eyes were closed, and he was in a deep coma. There were intravenous catheters (IVs) in his arms and an oxygen mask over his nose. His breathing was labored and noisy because of the fluid that had accumulated in his lungs. He was heavily sedated with morphine, which the medical staff felt was a merciful way of facilitating a less painful and more rapid exit from life. Because of congestion in his intestine, his abdomen had expanded like a huge balloon. I hung on to Peter's every breath, hoping it would not be his last.

My panic subsided when I felt an urgency to communicate with Peter in his deep inner state. Why did communication have to end just because he was not "talking" to us anymore? Both Arny and I felt that he was "there" and that, although he was in an altered state of consciousness, it was possible to cross the bridge to this foreign world.

Until this time, for many years, Arny had worked alone with people near death and in comatose states. Almost everyone in near-death conditions with whom Arny worked awakened in some form and told him amazing things. However, Arny hadn't spoken to anyone about what he witnessed because he was afraid that people would not believe some of the astonishing stories. Now, for the first time, he had a witness to what he had been experiencing.

Arny, Sandy, and I moved closer to the bed. We established connection with Peter by joining the rhythm of his breath. We did this by gently pressing his wrists in time with inhalation and exhalation. We noticed the minimal signals he gave: little twitches of fingers; alterations in his breathing from quick, shallow pants to deep breaths; sudden gasping sounds emanating from his lungs; and slight color changes in his face. We let Peter know that we were aware of his communications by commenting on these various signals. We encouraged him to follow and believe in the kinds of experiences that he was having and told him that his inner world would be our guide.

We held Peter's hands, and Peter slightly squeezed them. He made more sounds as we imitated the noises coming from his lungs. We could tell he was in contact with us, although we knew that the morphine injections subdued and delayed his communications.

After a couple of hours, when we were tired and needed to go to bed, I felt intuitively that something else was going to happen and that we shouldn't leave. Arny decided to pose the question to Peter, saying, "We have to work in our practices in the morning and need to get some sleep now. We need you to show us a greater signal of some sort or we, unfortunately, will have to go home."

What happened next reminded me of a riveting scene from a mummy movie I had seen as a kid. Peter, who had been lying more or less immobile for hours, immediately sat straight up in his bed. I remember the horrific crunching and cracking sound as this seemingly inanimate body suddenly bolted upright. Abruptly, Peter turned his head directly toward Arny and then just as suddenly lay down again! I almost fainted. Peter's wife gasped. Arny managed to say, "Hi!" Needless to say, we stayed.

Sandy asked the nurses not to give him another injection of morphine so that Peter could have more immediate connection with his inner experiences. The staff insisted that he was in pain and required the medication. We said that he did not appear to be in pain but was trying to communicate with us. His wife said that we had nothing to lose and should at least try. Finally the nurses agreed to delay the next injection.

As the night hours passed, we followed Peter's finger and leg movements and guttural sounds. Slowly he emerged from his coma into a more wakeful state. His very small finger motions increased, and his arms started to wave rhythmically in the air. As we joined his sound-making, his murmurings turned into coherent musical tones and then songs. He used his hands to conduct us as we joined him in singing and humming playful children's songs.

By morning Peter was sitting up in bed talking to us. His lungs had partially cleared. He was coughing a bit and complained that "the bottle is too small for the spirit inside." We were shocked by the use of such symbolic language because until this point, Peter was avidly against psychology or religion of any sort. We looked at Peter's stomach, a swollen vessel much too small for all the liquid it now contained. The spirit certainly was trapped in the body![5]

"That's no problem," Arny said. "Just take the cork out!" Peter queried, "Where is the cork?"—to which his body gave a somatic answer, a cough. Arny said, "The cork is in your throat. Just take it out!" Peter's eyes grew large and he started to smile. Suddenly he began to yelp and howl and cry and sing, making all sorts of sounds that were much too loud for the quiet nighttime atmosphere of the hospital ward. The spirit was out of the bottle and, shortly thereafter, his kidneys began to function again.

As time went on, Peter hugged all of us. He overflowed with loving words, reassuring us that everything was okay and that we would be all right. This man who had been so very shy was now speaking about love and eternity and was comforting us all. The nurses and doctors filed into the room and were shocked. Peter was supposed to have died the night before. Now he consoled the medical helpers and thanked them for their caring!

I remember feeling that I was in the presence of some saintly figure who not only miraculously arose out of his coma but became a teacher of love who healed everyone around him. Peter said that he was going to go on studying and, in the same breath, that we should look after his wife. The doctor who had told me that Peter would die that night came into the room. He faltered and looked shocked. He could only shake his head and say that what was happening could not be explained by medical science.

Finally, Arny and I had to go home to sleep. Later that day we heard that, after a party with his family, complete with the oranges and dark beer he had requested, and a healing interaction with Sandy, and after talking about love and life, Peter died peacefully and without symptoms in his sleep.

My Work

That night changed my life. I was stunned by the depth and possibilities of the human being, which were so much more astounding than I had ever thought possible. My only wish was that I could hold onto this realization and not sink back into ordinary life where dreams and inner experiences were of only fleeting importance. I realized that no matter what physical or psychological condition a person is in, that person is full of experiences and needs as much loving attention and sensitive communication as a person in what we think of as a "normal" state of consciousness. Although medical understanding of coma assumes that the comatose person is unaware and unresponsive, we found Peter traveling through meaningful inner states. By using communication methods adapted to Peter's altered state of consciousness, we were able to communicate with him and join him in a most amazing and moving journey. After expressing my feelings to Arny, we lit candles for Peter and thanked him for a most special teaching.

After this experience with Peter, Arny felt more empowered to write about his work with people in comatose states. In his book Coma[6] he tells Peter's tale, as well as other stories, and provides an inspirational thesis on the background, special meaning, and ethical implications of coma work. He focuses on coma work near death and provides the beginnings of coma work skills.

Since the publication of *Coma*, Arny and I have continued our work together. Over the past ten years, together with our colleagues, we have consulted and worked with doctors, nurses, and families helping people in comatose states all over the world. We have given coma work trainings for helping professionals and lay people and have provided advice over the phone to family members. Although Arny's work, as described in *Coma*, focused primarily on comatose conditions occurring near death, our work became increasingly involved with coma caused by brain injury.

A colleague, Stan Tomandl, published his manual, "Coma Work and Palliative Care," which provides an accessible introduction to process-oriented methods for work with the dying and people in remote states of consciousness.[7] Kay Ross has written an important article about her experiences as a registered nurse working with comatose patients, in which she compares our approach with coma patients to the medical/nursing methods typically applied.[8] *Coma, A Healing Journey* expands on these previous efforts and is intended as a comprehensive, step-by-step guide to coma work methods for all types of coma, including special methods necessary for working with people in comas caused by brain injury. It also offers introductory medical ideas about comas. (For more in-depth discussions of medical theory, see the Bibliography.) The information in this book is derived from our experiences with comatose people, from our workshops, and from my coma training classes.

The outcome of the coma methods I describe varies from patient to patient. Some comatose people awaken or partially awaken to tell amazing stories of their inner journeys, especially when the coma is due to near-death conditions. Sometimes people give feedback about their inner experiences and remain in the coma. Others are able to communicate with family members about their inner experiences. Some emerge from the coma and return to life; others find an entry into death. When assisting people in coma resulting from brain injury, coma methods also assist the natural recuperative process of the body. Responses may be slower as inner body connections embark on their recuperative journey. The person may become more "awake," but not yet be able to express herself in ordinary ways because of injuries to parts of the brain.

In each case, however, these methods help family, relatives, and caregivers to connect and communicate intimately with the comatose person. The comatose person is no longer isolated but feels related to and lovingly accompanied in her inner experiences.

Historical Overview of Coma

The word *coma* comes from the Greek *koma*, meaning "deep sleep, lethargy." Stories of the recognition of coma, and of experiences while in coma, have been passed down through the centuries.

Many accounts from different times and places tell of an individual's seeming death, release from the body, journeys to heaven, hell, or an afterlife of some sort, and then return. These experiences are often precipitated by injury, illness, dreaming, or ecstasy practices.[9] For example, at the end of *Republic*, Plato described the death of a soldier in battle and his return to life on the funeral pyre, after which he told onlookers of his journey to the other world.[10] Raising people from seeming "death" was attributed to Jesus on more than one occasion.

In the seventeenth century, a monk named Barontus was suddenly stricken by a fever and seemingly died but was actually comatose. After awakening he told of his journey to heaven and hell.[11] In the eighteenth and nineteenth centuries "it was recognized…that coma can imitate death and that people sometimes recover spontaneously from apparent death."[12]

To become a shaman in many native cultures, the initiate often goes through a comalike state in which he must have a close confrontation with and return from death, which is brought on by deliberate rituals or sudden illness.[13] The well-known story of Black Elk describes the experience of this Native American man, who went through a shamanic initiation at the age of nine.[14] Suddenly becoming paralyzed, Black Elk seemed to be dead. During that time he had many visions in which he was taken to the clouds and gained the gifts of spiritual insight and healing. He later returned to his tribe with visions of their future.

Today, coma is understood medically as a state much like sleep, in which individuals are completely unarousable and are unresponsive to external stimulation and to their inner needs.[15] Comas can be classified into the following broad categories:

1. Comas attributable to structural or mechanical injury.
2. Comas resulting from metabolic changes occurring near death or from insulin imbalances.
3. Comas with associated psychological or psychogenic factors that contribute to the comatose state.

In all three of these categories, people typically remain in the deepest level of coma for two to four weeks, then awaken, die, or enter into a slightly more wakeful, seemingly unresponsive state called a "persistent vegetative state." Especially in coma attributable to brain injury, as the recuperation process unfolds, many people may travel through various degrees of wakefulness during which they grow closer and closer to "the shores of awareness"[16] and everyday reality.

Currently, comatose patients are cared for in hospitals or other inpatient facilities, in rehabilitation centers for brain injury management, and, as a result of the hospice movement, at home. The Brain Injury Association in Washington, D.C. (originally called the National Head Injury Foundation), founded in 1980, was created to give support to and serve as an advocate for brain-injured individuals and their families.

Methods that have emerged for assisting comatose people, besides medical intervention, include the caretaker meditating or using imaginative techniques alongside the comatose person, and practices aimed at reawakening the senses and reorganizing brain pathways, such as coma arousal, multi-sensory stimulation and sensory integration, as well as ocean hyperbaric treatment in which pure oxygen is used in an attempt to revivify dormant cells of the brain.[17] Perhaps the most widespread method is a combination of love and hope.

In recent times, pioneers in the fields of near-death experience, work with the dying, bodywork, and work with altered states have helped us move toward a greater understanding of the deep states that comatose people may experience.[18]

Popular interest in the legal issues of coma cases soared in the United States in the 1970s and early 1980s in response to the trials in one of the first "right to die" cases, that of Karen Ann Quinlan. After the courts allowed life support to be removed, this young woman remained in a persistent vegetative state for nine years. Additional incidents point to the vital importance of further study concerning communicating with people in comatose conditions. Journalist Mary Kay Blakely, in her popular book, *Wake Me When It's Over*, described her experiences in and her emergence from a diabetic coma. The case of a young woman who was brutally beaten in Central Park in 1996 brought attention to the care of traumatically injured patients who are in coma and spotlighted the need for generally accepted standards of emergency procedures that could reduce the risk of further injury once the patient is admitted into the emergency room. A former editor of a well-known magazine, who suffered a stroke, emerged from his coma unable to communicate verbally, yet dictated an entire book about his inner experiences through blinks of an eyelid. In addition, excitement surged over a police officer emerging from what seemed to be a seven-and-a-half-year coma caused by a gunshot wound to the head.[19]

During the second half of the twentieth century, the entire process of death, once a taboo or hidden topic, particularly in Western culture, has surfaced (especially since the 1960s in the United States) as an unavoidable and important stage of life. The emergence of illnesses such as acquired immunodeficiency syndrome (AIDS) and cancer is a constant reminder of the care of seriously ill individuals, and has openly confronted many of us with the face of death. Elisabeth Kubler-Ross, a leader in the field of death and dying, raised our awareness of the stages of dying and grieving.[20] The modern hospice movement, with roots in medieval times, began in the 1960s in England as an alternative to hospital care for the dying.[21] Hospice is available when cure is no longer possible and is a patient- and family-directed program. It emphasizes the quality of life and palliative care rather than a cure-based approach.[22]

In the 1990s, numerous particular cases have brought attention to questions about an individual's choices and rights near death. In the United States, documents such as the "living will" have been drafted in which a person gives to a legal figure or family member the right to determine the withdrawal of artificial life support when death is imminent and the person, as a result of illness or injury, is incompetent to give an opinion.[23] By 1991, 40 states had affirmed the validity of some version of the living will (see Chapter 2 for more on this topic).

Also in the United States, the issue of "doctor-assisted suicide"—whether mentally competent, terminally ill patients have the right to obtain from a physician drugs that hasten death—has fired intense legal, religious, and moral debate. In 1994, a law was passed in Oregon approving doctor-assisted suicide.[24] This thorny public issue, which elicits strong emotions on each side of the debate, is beginning to appear on ballots in many parts of the country. In the 1990s, Dr. Jack Kevorkian has been on trial for being present at such deaths. In 1991, Derek Humphrey, founder of the Hemlock Society, published *Final Exit*, describing how terminally ill people can commit suicide, and the book topped best-seller lists.

All of these issues press us to develop ever more compassionate methods attuned to the quality of life and special needs of the dying person, which take into account more fully the person's desires concerning medication and health care, spiritual and emotional support, and choices concerning death. Yet, we face a great challenge to develop the ability not only to ask those who are able to "speak" for themselves, but also to ask—to give a vote to—those who are unable to communicate through ordinary means, that is, comatose people.

Until now, coma research has been weighted on the side of comas resulting from brain injury. Because of their frequency, predominance among young people, and tremendous emotional, social, and financial consequences, more effort is geared toward diagnosis and prediction of outcome for people in comas resulting from brain injury than for those in other forms of coma.[25] Also, it seems that comas resulting from brain injury allow family members more hope of recuperation and a willingness to try new methods. In contrast, comas that arise as a result of near-death conditions are rarely mentioned in the literature. In the Western world (until the recent developments cited above) it has been assumed that when someone is dying, all we can do is to make the person as comfortable as possible, take care of bodily needs, and create a warm and loving environment. While these activities are all essential, they are not the total picture. The dying process is also a potential stage of growth. In other regions of the world, such as Tibet and Egypt, death practices focus with great reverence on the dying process, a time seen to be filled with opportunity for consciousness.[26]

New Challenges

Recent advancements in medical technology have made it possible in some cases to keep someone alive longer than would have been possible even ten years ago. Yet, along with these remarkable developments, we are presented with new and serious difficulties. Vital functions can be maintained mechanically; at the same time, new and complex questions arise about the ethical and emotional issues concerning the continuance or discontinuance of life support, the type and extent of care for a person in a persistent vegetative state, where a person on life support should be cared for, long-term care issues associated with managed care in the United States, and insurance issues. Many of the people who survive brain injuries are between eighteen and twenty-four years of age, have vital young bodies, and may need long-term care. For families, frustration and anguish are further exacerbated by questions about the best form of care, insurance coverage, and moving the comatose person from site to site—not to mention the "baseline" trauma of the family resulting from the loved one's sudden coma, and their reliance on the predictions of medical staff about outcome.

Although far more people are in long-term vegetative states today than in the past, most caregivers know little more about how to communicate with these individuals than people knew centuries ago. Medical staff rarely have enough time to communicate effectually with a comatose person and—more to the point—are not trained in interacting with people in altered states of consciousness. This lack of training may stem from the prevalent viewpoint in the field of medicine, in which altered states of consciousness such as coma have not been understood as meaningful aspects of our experience. The comatose person is assumed to be unconscious and unaware. In general, modern medical interventions for coma emphasize the importance of focusing on sustaining life and arousing people from the comatose state. If the person does not awaken or does not respond to questions, the situation is sometimes viewed as a medical failure, a factor further depressing everyone involved.

Currently we do not have methods of communicating with someone in this state and helping that person follow her inner experiences. Because we are unable to communicate directly with her, no one is ever really certain about the comatose person's wishes. This results in greater stress and agony for all. An updated training must include special methods geared toward sensitively communicating with the person in this all-too-frequent state of consciousness. We have been encouraged by positive feedback from professional caregivers who have applied our coma methods successfully.

The advent of home hospice care has reminded us of the possibility of creating a warmer, more intimate environment for those in the last stages of life, many of whom may fall into a coma at some point. Hospice care helpers offer loving support and care; yet, family members and friends may be unprepared for—and afraid of—a home-based hospice situation. Most of us are unaccustomed to being with people who are in comatose states or near-death conditions. If you are assisting a loved one who is in a comatose state, in addition to the medical issues, you also must contend with pressing personal concerns, such as feeling fearful and uncertain about being with someone who is in a coma, perhaps suffering anguish yourself about your loved one who is "hanging on" so long. Even basic questions can tax you: "Should I stay in the room all the time?" "Will she ever wake up?" "How can I communicate with him now that he is so far away?" "Can the person hear me?" "How do I deal with the possible death of this person I love?"

We ponder unfinished relationship issues, religious beliefs, family ties and separations, hopes of recovery, or relief from pain. Much of our distress comes about because we do not know what the person in coma is experiencing.

A Process Approach to Comatose States: A Path with Heart

The process-oriented view of comatose states is that they are due to mechanical and chemical problems and that they reflect deep, altered states of consciousness in which the person is going through potentially meaningful inner experiences. We do not focus on the comatose person solely from the viewpoint of pathology—that the person is ill and must be healed—but from a phenomenological viewpoint. That is, we observe and try to assist the person's inner experiences. People do not operate as simply as machines that can break down and be repaired; people are full of potential growth in all states of consciousness—even up to and perhaps beyond the moment of death. Some people in coma may be unconsciously searching for the chance to go deeply inside without the disturbances of, or having to relate to, everyday life. In coma work we assume that if the heart is still beating, we should make the attempt to communicate and not rule out the possibility of reaching these little-known corners of life.

Comatose individuals inevitably appreciate the assistance of someone who is able to relate to them in special ways and who lovingly assists them in following and unfolding inner experiences. Coma work makes it possible for individuals in coma to communicate with a helper if they like, and to have a voice in decisions about their care.

I remember a particularly moving case Arny told me about. He was working with a six-year-old European boy who had a brain tumor and had fallen into a coma. The boy was expected to die very soon. Arny used special communication methods he had developed to ask the boy yes-and-no questions and receive answers. Arny had noticed that the skin on the boy's cheeks would sometimes turn very red. Arny set up a communication system: when the skin became very red, this meant yes. When there was no color change, the answer was no. He asked the boy a number of basic children's questions:

"Are you in a coma because you hate your brother and sister?"

No response.

"Are you in a coma because you don't want to go to school?"

No response.

After exhausting many possibilities, Arny asked his last question:

"Are you in a coma because you want to be closer to God?"

The little boy's cheeks grew bright red.

At that point the father said, "No! He cannot become a priest!"

What a shock! Arny asked the parents to step outside so he could continue to discuss with the child his religious desires. Later, he talked with the parents about their opposition to their son becoming a priest. A number of weeks later, Arny heard that the child had come out of the coma, and today he is studying theology at a university.

Process-oriented coma work does not focus on getting the person to awaken, although this sometimes happens, particularly in near-death conditions. The goal is to communicate with the comatose person and provide a loving sense of companionship. Once this connection is fostered, the helper will have the chance of helping the comatose person follow and unfold his inner experiences. Coma methods make it possible to ask the comatose person questions and take into consideration his wishes. When brain injury is involved, coma methods also assist the person's natural recuperative process.

This is a path with heart, a path that values all levels and dimensions of human life. It focuses on following nature, that is, appreciating the person's unique process.

Note: The special communication methods described in this manual should be used only after all medical emergencies have been relieved as much as possible.

At the edge of death and in the throes of coma as a result of brain injury, many people, like Peter, go through deep experiences that express universal or mythic themes such as climbing mountains, meeting a lover, engaging in a battle, traveling to new territory, reaching for the stars, discovering aspects of the meaning of their lives, or getting in contact with experiences they have intuited their whole lives.

For example, an elderly man who had had a stroke revealed to us during his coma, through responses to yes-and-no questions, that he was climbing a mountain and meeting a woman. A young comatose boy who was hit by a car told us, through physical responses to our verbal and movement-oriented communication, that he was in the middle of a great heroic battle. Ross writes about a young girl who came out of her coma and reported that she had been to a lovely holiday place where she didn't have to do what she was told.[27] It seems that people, no matter what their state of consciousness, are always striving to know and become themselves.

Some people "hang on" at the end of life to complete "unfinished business." We recently visited a woman who had cancer and was in a coma, very near death. In her ordinary life this woman had not been prone to expressing emotions. Her husband was shy about our coming to see his wife because he did not know us and because of this sensitive and intimate moment. But he felt his wife had something else to do before she died and that was why she was still alive. It was a very difficult time for him, partly because he did not know how best to communicate with her or to find out what she was experiencing.

After Arny and I worked with her for a brief period, the woman, who was heavily sedated with morphine, began to squeeze our hands as a way of showing that she was present and that she had something to complete. The next day we heard that shortly after we had left, the woman awakened from her coma, gathered her whole family around, and told them how much she loved them. She died peacefully the day after expressing this message.

Learning to Communicate with Comatose People

Coma work requires an ability to expand our normal ways of communicating because the comatose person cannot talk to us in an ordinary manner. It requires that we learn to relate to the person's altered state. If we adjust our communication style to the comatose person's world, we have always been able—in some form—to reach the person in coma. The most sensitive people seem to do this kind of communication naturally. Even if you do not know many skills, a comatose person responds well to loving attention in which you try to join in and adapt your communication style to the altered state of the comatose person.

I recall a young mother accompanying her ten-year-old son, who was comatose as a result of brain injury. This woman was extremely loving. She gently touched her son's forehead, talked near his ear in a very intimate way, and laid her head lightly on his chest. Almost instantly, the boy began to react, turning his face toward her and murmuring sounds. Her gentle, sensitive way of interacting bridged a seemingly endless abyss.

Many people talk to comatose patients as if they were in a "normal" awake state of consciousness. Relatives and friends want so badly for the person in coma to look at them, chat with them, sit up, and relate as if they were the person before the coma. In other instances, a person's bodily needs may be attended to, but little more. Sometimes the comatose person may be assumed to be, in essence, blind, deaf, and mute. All of these reactions are quite normal. Most of us cannot understand or fathom why someone isn't talking in an ordinary way anymore. It seems that without ordinary means of communicating, the person just can't be there. Many people are surprised by the types of communication the comatose person may make, including sounds, small gestures, or even movements, which seem so different from the way we communicate in ordinary reality. It is difficult for many of us to realize that someone we love is in a different state of consciousness, that this person is present but requires special methods of communication. However, many parents and close friends sense that the person is present and can be connected with.

Once Arny and I were working with a comatose patient who had been in a car accident and was lying in an urban hospital. In the next bed there was a twenty-five-year-old man who had come out of his coma but was still in a somewhat dreamy state. Instead of talking in a clear way when the nurses spoke to him, he would vaguely nod in recognition of their presence and then drift off and begin to speak ecstatically about music. "Johnny, what day is it?" they persisted. Johnny replied, "That music is so beautiful." "Johnny, look at the calendar," they said. "Do you know what day it is? What time it is?" Johnny replied, "Do you hear it?"

While the nurses wanted Johnny to return to a "normal" state of consciousness, Johnny was in the middle of another process. He needed someone to join him in his inner world. Our experience has shown that when people in such twilight states of consciousness feel understood, they more easily return to ordinary reality.

Coma training classes have made one challenge quite clear. I have noticed that the majority of class participants feel uncomfortable relating to someone in an altered state of consciousness. Typically students sit far away from the comatose person, looking frozen, terrified, and uptight. It is as though a huge abyss separates the helper from the person receiving the help. No matter how many times I encourage people to get closer, it doesn't help. Behind this awkwardness lie fears about relating to someone in a different state of consciousness from our own, and also personal issues about intimacy and physical contact. I pondered how to create a bridge and have found the techniques in this book to be of great help.

Thus it became apparent that it is not sufficient to teach people the skills by which they can assist a comatose patient. Attention must also be placed on the helper's personal psychology and development, particularly in relation to altered states, feelings about life and death, and the degree of comfort with the use of touch, sound, and movement as communication tools.

Although physicians are aware that people seem to have strong dreams or images and experiences during comas, this area is little explored and is assumed to result solely from chemical changes in the brain.[28] Consider this statement from well-known Swedish poet Artur Lundkvist, about his experience in a coma resulting from a heart attack:

> I know I am travelling all the time, possibly with no interruptions, also with no tremors or noises, soundlessly and softly, and then I am no longer lying in my bed but stepping out into the world where everything is awake, sundrenched, comforting, and I am there clearly as a visitor, and I am quite at ease.[29]

While to the outside observer Lundkvist seemed to be in a "vacant," unaware state, he reveals to us a deep inner world of experiences.

Maggie Callanan and Patricia Kelley, two nurses who work with the dying, remind us of the necessity of appreciating non-ordinary states of consciousness and symbolic communications of dying people. Some of these people are labeled "confused" or "disoriented" and their communications are misunderstood because they are symbolic and seemingly obscure. Callanan and Kelley suggest that "by keeping open minds and by listening carefully to dying people, we can begin to understand messages they convey through symbol or suggestion."[30]

As we learn more about the special needs of those who are ill or close to death, we must also develop more humane methods of caring for and communicating with those in comatose states. Coma work means learning a new language, learning to communicate through sounds, visions, breath, feeling, and movement. By doing so, we bridge the gap between the ordinary world and the world of those who seem so far away. In this way, we join these comatose persons, giving them a chance to express their innermost wishes and selves.

Notes

1. Multi-Society Task Force on the PVS, "Medical Aspects of PVS: Statement of the Multi-Society Task Force. Part I," 1503.
2. Fahrlaender, "Medizinische, Rechtliche und Ethische Probleme bei Permanentem Vegetativem Zustand," 1191–1195.
3. Frankowski, Annegers, and Whitman, "Epidemiological and Descriptive Studies. Part I," 33–43.
4. Gilfix, Gilfix, and Sinatra, "The Persistent Vegetative State," 63–71.
5. Arny Mindell, (*Dreambody*) calls this phenomenon the "dreambody"; the mirror experience between dream imagery and body experiences.
6. Arnold Mindell, *Coma: The Dreambody Near Death.*
7. Tomandl, *Coma Work and Palliative Care.*
8. Ross, "A Comparison of the Medical/Nursing and Process Work Approaches to Coma," 23–31.
9. Zaleski, *Otherworld Journeys,* 45.
10. Ibid., 19.
11. Ibid., 45. In the eighteenth century, tales of the dead suddenly awakening spread fear of premature burial and contributed to the development of new laws about burial practices. Also, more than 200 years ago the first Humane Society in Amsterdam arose as a result of the realization that some people who have drowned can be revived through certain methods. Technology for resuscitation bloomed in the 1950s (President's Commission, *Defining Death,* 12).
12. Ivan and Ventureyra, "Coma and the Evolution of Brain Resuscitation in Coma," 5.
13. Zaleski, *Otherworld Journeys,* 13.
14. Neidhardt, *Black Elk Speaks.*
15. Clayman, ed., *American Medical Association Encyclopedia of Medicine,* 294.
16. A phrase used by Jean-Dominique Bauby in his *The Diving Bell and the Butterfly,* in which he tells about his experience of "locked-in" syndrome resulting from a stroke in which his mind was fully intact but he was able to communicate solely through the blink of an eyelid.
17. See Roger La Borde's work, discussed in "Back From Coma" by Brad Lemley (80–82), for meditative and imaginative methods; see

also Michael Kearney's *Mortally Wounded,* on imagery work with individuals who are dying but not in comatose states. See Edward LeWinn's *Coma Arousal,* in which the use of intense, continual stimulus to reawaken the senses is discussed as well as the work of the Institutes for the Achievement of Human Potential and Glenn Doman, Roselise Wilkinson, Mihai D. Dimancescu and Ralph Pelligran's article, "The Effect of Intense Multi-sensory Stimulation on Coma Arousal and Recovery"; see also Beverly Slater's *Coping With Head Injury* (153–154) on sensory integration, a method used in cases of brain injury to improve the person's senses according to developmental lines, and the Discovery Channel television program "Coma: The Silent Epidemic," on the use of intensive stimulation of undamaged parts of brain to take over damaged ones. There is debate in the medical community about the usefulness of such sensory stimulation techniques. Ocean hyperbaric treatment is also mentioned in the Discovery Channel program just cited.

18. Pioneers in the field of near-death experiences include Raymond Moody, Elisabeth Kubler-Ross, and Kenneth Ring; in working with the dying see Kubler-Ross, Stephen and Ondrea Levine, Maggie Callanan and Patricia Kelley, and the work of the Zen Hospice Project. For more on bodywork see Aminah Raheem, Fritz Smith, and Andrea Olsen. On altered states see most notably the writings of Charles Tart. (See the Bibliography for references to specific works of these authors.)

19. On Karen Ann Quinlan see Joseph and Julie Quinlan's *Karen Ann: The Quinlans Tell Their Story.* On the woman beaten in Central Park in 1996, see Malcolm Gladwell's "Conquering the Coma"; in addition, see the PBS television program "Coma" for more on the new standards for emergency care for head trauma, which were approved by the World Health Organization on May 15, 1997. On the editor of *Elle* magazine who had a stroke, see Bauby, *The Diving Bell and the Butterfly.* On the policeman who emerged from coma, see Tim Friend's article "Seeking Clear-headed Conversation About Coma." In subsequent review of the latter case, some physicians have questioned whether the man was ever in a true coma. This man awoke from his "coma," spoke to his family, seemed to slip back into the coma, and died a year later. Whatever the case may be, the general public seems intrigued by the stories of such states.

20. See, for example, Kubler-Ross, *On Death and Dying.*

21. Taylor, *The Hospice Movement in Britain,* 5–6.

22. George Young, "Hospice and Health Care."

23. Betty A. Prashker, ed., *The Columbia University College of Physicians and Surgeons Complete Home Medical Guide,* 54–55.

24. Mark O'Keefe, "Voters' Guide to Measure 51: Doctor Assisted Suicide Repeal," *The Oregonian* (Portland), October 19, 1997, A20.

25. Plum and Posner, *The Diagnosis of Stupor and Coma,* 330.

26. For example, see Sogyal Rinpoche's *The Tibetan Book of Living and Dying.*

27. Ross, "A Comparison of the Medical/Nursing and Process Work Approaches to Coma," 28.

28. David Ingvar, MD, states, "We do not know why our brains begin to manufacture images and impressions of sights and sounds—even music after we have experienced lack of oxygen or altered ventilation in our bodies…There is very little control over what happens to the psyche. The same phenomenon, although to a much lesser degree, occurs during normal sleep." Quoted in Artur Lundkvist's, *Journeys in Dream and Imagination,* 8–9.

29. Lundkvist, *Journeys in Dream and Imagination,* 23.

30. Callanan and Kelley, *Final Gifts,* 14.

T schierv is a very old, small, quiet mountain town in Switzerland, embedded high in the Alps, close to the Italian border. To reach it is a constant challenge, as many of the mountain passes suddenly close because of danger of avalanche from heavy snowfall. In that isolated, age-old village, a group of process work students took part in a "deep bodywork and religious experience" seminar given by Arny. We all stayed in a very rustic stone house. The floors and walls of the seminar room were made of large stones that grew cold as night fell, yet the atmosphere of excitement, research, and discovery made it seem like we were always by a cozy, warm fire. We spent a couple of weeks exploring our own deep body states. We cooked our meals on a wood stove and stayed up all hours of the night talking, dancing, working, and philosophizing.

It was there in Tschierv that I learned most about how deep, meaningful processes lie just below the surface in people's bodies. Special hands-on bodywork methods made it possible to access experiences that helped me remember my whole self. I recall one exercise we did on trance states. My helper lifted my arm so slowly and gently,

in such a subtle way, that I found myself falling into a deep trance and remained there for quite a long time. I remember journeying through a very spiritual vision in which I felt that I was witnessing Jesus curing the lepers. This vision was a source of comfort and guidance for me.

I remember that vision each time I hold the hand of a person in a coma and follow her breathing. I remember that she, too, may be going through a spiritual experience of unique value to her. Many people in comatose states and near-death conditions are freed from their ordinary identities and often undergo mythic or spiritual peak experiences, or both.[1]

What Is Ordinary?

Let's think about our ordinary or normal state of consciousness in detail. What is considered ordinary or normal is culturally defined. Let's say that a normal state of consciousness is one in which a person is able to function reasonably well. She can adapt to everyday life by responding when someone talks to her, smiling when appropriate, acting wide awake when she is supposed to, getting to places on time, and so forth.

An altered state of consciousness is any alteration from this ordinary state of consciousness. Coma is the deepest of altered states in which a person seemingly does not react to outer stimuli and is apparently not able to communicate in any way.

Altered states are really not that unfamiliar to us. All of us experience degrees of altered states throughout the day. Just remember those times when your attention wanders, when you are thrilled about the new dog you just got, in a passionate embrace, sexually aroused, utterly "spaced out," tired, or falling into deep meditation. Many of us know about altered states from drug or alcohol experiences, severe bouts of illness, or strong emotional states when we are brimming with anger or deeply in love and seem to "lose ourselves." We seek altered states when we go to movies or listen to music to temporarily shift out of our ordinary frame of mind. Just waking up in the morning sleepy, in a confused or dreamy state, is perhaps the most common example. If someone tries to pull you out of this twilight consciousness, you probably feel annoyed and misunderstood.

Often we do not accord any value to these common forms of altered states. We've learned to push them to the side. We say, "It was nothing," "I was only fantasizing," or "I was just upset" to explain an extraordinary behavior or response. Yet, none of us wants to be glued permanently to ordinary reality! Human nature is much too creative to remain in only one mode of being. We tend to foster the idea that altered states are insignificant and carry this viewpoint to more extreme forms of altered states such as coma.

Shamans and healers throughout time have consciously gone into altered-state trances for healing purposes.[2] If we investigate our own altered states, we can discover the beginnings of meaningful inner processes and self-healing abilities knocking at our door, requesting that we open up to other aspects of ourselves.

Not long ago I came down with a high fever while we were traveling, and I prayed that we would get home so I could go to bed. I just wanted the sick feeling to end. For a week I was too ill and feverish to do much but lie down. I had a serious case of flu. I was miserable at first, whining, sweating, and unable to get comfortable.

One evening as I was lying in bed, I realized that I was drifting in and out of consciousness and that I actually was beginning to enjoy my light-headed, drowsy condition. It was an absolute relief from my intensely packed days. I felt empty, at ease, and unencumbered. I realized a part of me wanted to stay in that far-out state, safe from the demands of daily life. Getting better would mean that I would lose contact with this inner tranquillity, which allowed me to stay close to myself.

I fell asleep and dreamed of a comatose man lying in bed. Someone had forgotten to put up the side rails. In his coma, the man turned over and fell out of bed, hit his head on the floor, and suffered another brain injury! He was in a double coma, so to speak. When I "woke up" to the meaning of my own illness, I realized how much I needed that empty-headed state and wanted to bring it into my life as a whole instead of ignoring it and going back to the way life was. Altered states can be very important!

The Caretaker's Altered States

For those of us in caretaker roles, knowledge of our own altered states is crucial because without this, we can feel quite uncomfortable trying to relate to someone else who is in a deep coma. All too easily we find ourselves wanting the comatose person to relate in a "normal" way instead of appreciating and following the altered state that the comatose person is in. We have found that the kinds of experiences comatose people have are not that different from the altered-state experiences we go through all the time, though typically in less dramatic form.

Knowing our own altered states has important implications, not only for assisting comatose people but for our personal lives as well. Much of our fear of dying has to do with the fear of being trapped by internal states we cannot control. By exploring our own altered states and our inner worlds while in seemingly good health, we can prepare for altered states that we may find ourselves in later in life. I remember a colleague who recently died. During his life he had spent a lot of time following and discovering his altered-state experiences. In his last moments of life, he seemed to make an easy, conscious transition into death, probably because of his earlier practices.

Without openness to our own altered states, we may have a tendency to marginalize people who do not fit into the communication norms of our culture. Hyperactive or withdrawn children, mentally challenged individuals, people in extreme psychotic states are looked upon as sick or disturbing. When we relegate people to such labels we never really learn how to communicate outside a very narrow range. We assume that the actions of these people are chaotic or meaningless, and do not challenge ourselves to understand their worlds.[3]

Coma and Medical Theory

Traditional definitions of coma in neurological journals are based on the following:

1. Cause-and-effect factors: what caused the coma and how it has affected the individual.
2. Consciousness and outcome: the degree of consciousness and subsequent prognosis or outcome.[4]

The American Medical Association defines coma as:

> …a state of unconsciousness and unresponsiveness distinguishable from sleep in that the person does not respond to external stimulation (i.e., shouting, pinching) or to his or her inner needs (i.e., full bladder). Coma results from disturbance or damage to areas of the brain, mostly cerebrum and upper parts of brain stem, involved in conscious activity or maintenance of consciousness.[5]

The definition of coma also states that during coma there is a lack of the sleep/wake cycle.

In general, coma onset is often associated physically with increased pressure in the brain that is due to changes in the brain tissue, blood, or cerebrospinal fluid. Pressure interferes with brain functioning and may cause the death of brain cells. Emergency medical procedures that relieve the pressure are imperative to prevent further deterioration of the brain. Unconsciousness is a result of swelling that presses on the reticular activation system.[6]

According to literature, three of the most commonly named causes of comatose states are alcoholism, stroke, and trauma (in that order). In children coma is most often caused by physical trauma or complications resulting from a tumor or seizures.[7] (Note: This medical list of common causes of coma does not include, or mention the frequency of, coma that is due to metabolic changes occurring near death. In fact, that type of coma is rarely discussed in the literature except for the mention of vegetative states which some people fall into as a result of degenerative diseases.) In evaluating coma in different levels of brain function doctors try to locate abnormalities and, from this standpoint, determine treatment and possible outcome.

As noted in Chapter 1, generally the deepest level of coma lasts from two to four weeks (sometimes longer in children, especially after trauma). Emerging from this deepest form of coma, the person may enter into a long-term state in which she appears awake but is unresponsive and in which the sleep/wake cycle returns. This state is variously called akinetic mutism, vegetative state, apallic syndrome, or coma vigil. One or both eyes remain open but with seeming lack of responsiveness to outer stimuli and an apparent lack of cognitive functioning. New research has begun to differentiate between a persistent and a permanent vegetative state depending on the time frame (see later discussion in this chapter). Some doctors restrict the use of the term *coma* to include only those states which resemble sleep and in which the eyes remain closed, although there is as yet no agreement about this.

When a person emerges further from a coma he may pass through a range of states of consciousness. These conditions are categorized medically by the degree of awareness the person appears to have. Some of these states include clouding of consciousness, delirium, and stupor,[8] locked-in syndrome, and the minimally responsive state.[9] People recuperating from brain injury may pass through stages of readjustment in which they experience varying degrees of limitation (or recovery) of various bodily and mental functions. In a sense they are straddling the worlds between a strongly altered state and ordinary consciousness.

For ease, in this book I refer to all of these states as coma. We work with people regardless of the various names and descriptions of the state of consciousness or diagnosis, focusing, rather, phenomenologically on the person's inner experiences and behavior.

Consciousness: Behavior or Awareness

Medically, the term *consciousness* is defined as a "state of awareness of the self and the environment." It includes the "ability to discriminate among both the sensory inputs and the internal cognitive aspects," as well as "wakefulness or alertness to external and internal processes."[10] Coma is defined as the extreme opposite: the comatose person is completely unresponsive and not arousable or "there is no psychologically understandable response to external stimuli or inner needs."[11]

While the traditional view of consciousness is adequate for certain purposes, it is limited by the perception of behavior as assessed by an outside observer. It relies on what an observer is able to notice about the comatose person's behavior and responsiveness to his inner needs and outer environment within the observer's frame of reference. The Multi-Society Task Force on Persistent Vegetative States (PVS) states that:

> ...there is...a biologic limitation to the certainty of this [medical] definition [of consciousness], since we can only infer the presence or absence of conscious experience in another person.... Thus, it is theoretically possible that a patient who appears to be in a vegetative state retains awareness but shows no evidence of it.[12]

Young, Blume, and Lynch[13] describe tests given to determine cognitive processes by the delivery of a question and the observation of a response. Yet, they say, it is very difficult to exclude that cognition or the possibility of cognition exists, that thought processes can occur even if they do not manifest through overt outer behavior:

> It is possible to determine that an individual is capable of thought if he responds purposefully to stimulation, but we cannot conclusively demonstrate that cognitive processes are not going on in the absence of such behavior.[13]

They continue:

> Thought, at its most basic level is obvious only to the individual; clinically, we cannot adequately assess the dysfunction of this most highly prized brain activity.[14]

In addition, Plum and Posner tell us that "the limits of consciousness are hard to define satisfactorily and quantitatively and we can only infer the self-awareness of others by their appearance and by their acts." They add that "psychologic factors can influence behavior as much as physiologic ones and usually require different medical management."[15]

Because of these uncertainties, we must leave open the possibility (and many people are becoming aware of this) that our current knowledge of how to elicit responses from individuals in an altered state, how to make contact with their inner experiences, and how to interpret responses may be limited by our lack of training and understanding of altered states of consciousness. Viewed only through the eyes of ordinary reality and "ordinary" responses, we may miss a comatose person's inner world of dreams and experiences. A recent study published in the *British Medical Journal* found that some people who have been labeled vegetative have been aware but unable to make contact in ordinary ways.[16] A paralyzed person, for example, may be awake and alert, yet unable to make himself understood by others.

It is quite natural, because of the manner in which many people have learned to communicate, to assume that comatose persons are "not there" if they do not respond to our questions in a way that we expect or are accustomed to. However, the communication of people in altered states of consciousness is frequently different from our ordinary modes of behavior.

All of us know what it is like to tune out questions we are asked when we are involved in something else and do not want to be distracted. Much of the time we end up ignoring what the person says and try to go on with what we are doing. Many of us know the experience of being in a foreign country where we have interpreted a particular gesture to mean one thing when it has a totally different meaning in that culture. Similarly, we should be careful not to assume that someone who doesn't answer a request for a response in the way we are accustomed to be answered is necessarily unavailable, or that the types of signals the person communicates, which we do not understand, are meaningless. That person may be relating from a very different kind of inner experience, and special types of communication and understanding may be required.

Therefore another way of understanding the potential for consciousness in comatose states is to view the state from the comatose person's *inner* awareness. Consider this analogy. Imagine that you go up to someone's house and look in the window. You see someone doing very strange postural things, like putting one foot behind her head. From the outside, you think, "This person has lost it!" But if you go inside the house, you find out that the person is actually practicing yoga! Her actions are not meaningless. Often we can only understand what the person is doing (or not doing) if we go inside and find out about her inner world.

As long as the heart is still beating, and even if the person is receiving mechanical ventilation ("on a ventilator"), we do not rule out the possibility that the potential for awareness exists. Most important, we should take into account both our observations of the behaviors of comatose people as these relate to ordinary criteria of consciousness and the assessment of consciousness by connecting with and valuing inner experiences and this special type of awareness.[17] We have found that comatose individuals do communicate and respond when they are related to in special ways that are adapted to their altered states and inner experiences.

Different Types of Comas

As touched on in Chapter 1, for the purpose of this manual the definition of coma is widened to include three ways of differentiating comas from a therapeutic viewpoint. These are: comas resulting from structural brain injury; from metabolic changes; or from psychogenic factors. Coma may be a result of some combination of these, or one of these causes can lead to the others. All of the practical methods described in this book can be used with all three types of comas, including their various stages. Some methods are specifically geared toward working with people who have suffered from structural brain injury and subsequent stages of recuperation (see Chapters 6, 12, and 13).

Structural comas result from mechanical damage to the brain attributable to traumatic or non-traumatic sources. Traumatic sources include accidents or acts of violence, which in turn may lead to blood clots in the brain stem, strokes, hemorrhages, or local impairment in blood flow. Non-traumatic sources of brain injury include abnormalities such as brain tumors and abscesses, inflammations, and metabolic or anoxic changes that result in structural damage to the brain. Examples of these metabolic and anoxic changes include hypoxia or anoxia in which there is an impaired blood flow to areas of the brain as a result of cardiac or respiratory arrest, birth complications, near-drowning, drug overdose, alcoholism, electric shock, prolonged convulsions, or poisoning.[18]

Our use of the term *metabolic coma* refers to a condition arising in response to changes in blood chemistry that result in a general reduction of the bodily function but that has not developed to the point of causing structural damage to the brain. Metabolic comas occur when the chemical balance of body fluids is severely disrupted for a critical period of time. This occurs in conditions such as diabetes, when the insulin/glucose balance is not regulated, or in near-death states, when the sodium/potassium balance is disrupted.[19] Drug overdose and alcoholism are also potential causes of metabolic comas.

Hospice and medical personnel associate the metabolic type of coma with near-death conditions and a gradual slowing down of body functions. The body is run down, but the brain is not injured. People in metabolic comas "usually suffer from partial dysfunction affecting many levels of the neuraxis simultaneously, yet concurrently retain the integrity of other functions originating at the same levels."[20]

In general, structural comas are less reversible and harder to recuperate from than metabolic comas. When structural damage has occurred, more rebuilding and healing of physical tissue must occur. Depending on the cause, metabolic comas can be more reversible and the chance of cognitive restoration is greater.

Injury or disturbance to the brain can originate from local or diffuse causes or from a combination of both. Local injury refers to trauma that has occurred at a particular area of the brain and can cause correspondingly specific defects in mental or motor functioning, such as loss of coordination, difficulty with speech, or paralysis. For example, when particular motor functions of the brain are affected, "decorticate posturing" frequently occurs in which the hands and fingers of the comatose person are rigidly bent in and upward toward the heart. Diffuse injury occurs when poisonous substances accumulate and intoxicate tissue in many areas of the brain. This type of injury can result from drug overdose, advanced liver or kidney disease, acute alcoholic intoxication, an infection of the brain such as encephalitis, or uncontrolled diabetes mellitis, in which the body is chronically unable to burn up ingested sugars. The most important diffuse cause is prolonged cerebral hypoxia.[21]

Psychogenic coma refers to coma in which organic reasons for the coma have been removed or healed but the person remains comatose for no known reason. This continuance of coma may be psychogenically or psychologically based. Such factors as mania or depression can contribute to this comatose condition. Sometimes these psychogenic factors are present before the onset of coma, although there are no statistics about this correlation.[22] Yet, we should be aware that, in essence, psychogenic or psychological factors accompany every comatose state.

To imagine what it is like to have a head injury, envision "waking up in a house where all the furniture has been rearranged and some of it is missing. The house is the same, but it's hard to get used to the new arrangement."[23] Aspects of our environment are familiar, but we are disoriented by the changes in the house and are unable to adapt readily.

Another metaphor: Arny describes the experience of a brain-injured comatose person as being in the driver's seat of her car, but the wires of the car aren't connected. The person tries to turn the steering wheel, but the wheels don't move. In contrast, the person in a metabolic coma is in a fully or partly operational car that is somewhat run down. The driver of the car is spaced out, or sleepy, or is just about to get out of the car. The person in a coma with underlying psychogenic factors is in a car that may have had any of the above difficulties, depending on the origins of the comatose state. However, even when the car is once again fully functioning, the driver is no longer interested in driving it. For example, this may be the case with depression.

Tests, Assessment, and Predictions

When someone is in a coma, various tests are used to identify the kind of brain disturbance that has occurred. Electrical activity within the brain can be tested with an electroencephalogram (EEG). The EEG is used to determine if the person is alert, awake, or asleep. A computerized tomography (CT) or computerized axial tomography (CAT) scan and magnetic resonance imaging (MRI) reveal physical abnormalities through high-quality, cross-sectional views of body tissues. The CT scan uses a combination of computer and x-ray technology. The MRI does not use x-rays or other irradiation and generally provides more contrast between normal and abnormal tissues than the CT scan.

In general, a comatose person fares best when treatment is received as quickly as possible. The most expeditious recovery takes place during the first six months.[24] If the time spent in coma after a brain injury is brief, it is likely that the person will recover full or nearly full function. When the time spent in coma lengthens, problems with physical and mental abilities are more common.[25] By and large, people with brain injury resulting from trauma have a better prognosis for consciousness than do those who have suffered brain injury as a result of oxygen deficiency. As a whole, children seem to have better prognoses.[26]

According to medicine, in less severe cases the person in coma may respond to stimulation by uttering a few words or moving an arm. More severe cases are indicated by apparent failure to respond to repeated vigorous stimuli. But deeply comatose people may show some autonomic reflex responses—such as unaided breathing, coughing, yawning, blinking, or roving eye movements—which indicate that the lower brain stem is still functioning. A person with no apparent activity in the cerebrum can remain alive for years because the brain stem is functioning. Spread of damage to lower brain stem may impair vital functions.[27]

The best medical method for charting and predicting the course of events in coma conditions is a well-documented formal neurological evaluation. Two methods for charting and predicting the course of coma, as assessed by a person's response to outer stimuli, are the Glasgow Coma Scale and the Rancho Los Amigos Scale of Cognitive Functioning.

The Glasgow Coma Scale[28] establishes the level of consciousness of the brain-injured person. The patient is scored on a scale of one to fifteen. The scale classifies verbal, motor, and eye-opening responses to outer stimulation. A high score indicates a better prognosis; a lower score corresponds to more severe damage to the brain and a worse prognosis for recovery.

The Rancho Los Amigos Scale of Cognitive Functioning[29] charts the stages of recovery of brain-injured individuals. Its scale ranges from "no response" in connection with outer stimuli, to "generalized response" in which the person gives inconsistent and seemingly non-purposeful responses, to "more appropriate but confused" behavior. The optimal state is "purposeful and appropriate" behavior, in which the person is oriented in time and space and can begin to function in and respond to the outer environment.

Medical staff monitor scores on these scales for signs of improvement or degeneration of the comatose state. These scores may determine the patient's treatment—whether he can remain in a particular medical facility, whether he is considered brain dead, the amount of resource allocation to allow for his treatment, or whether he should be transferred to a different facility with greater or lesser duration and intensity of care (depending on the views of medical staff and insurance companies). These tests, however, rely once again on the observations of an outside observer rather than eliciting the comatose person's inner experiences.

Further unanswered questions about the methodology of such tests include variations in how to ask questions, how much repetition and duration is necessary, what the size of response must be, what to make of responses that occur without stimulus, who should give the tests, what to do if family members receive responses and the doctors do not, and so on.

It should be remembered that brain injury affects every person differently. Prediction is difficult. No one really understands why a person may recover and build new nerve cells, when for weeks it has looked as if she would die or remain in a vegetative state. It is also intriguing to notice that the severity of impairment cannot always be directly correlated with the severity of impact to the head.

Still, most doctors concur that, medically speaking, the potential recuperation of people who have had structural brain injury requires a great deal of time in order for the body to restore, heal, and reconstruct nerve cells, synapses, leaking capillaries, and other vital parts of the brain. The difficulty in making definitive prognoses, combined with the extended length of recovery (particularly from brain injury), can be quite distressing for family and friends.

Persistent versus Permanent Vegetative State

Current research aimed at better prognosis attempts to define even clearer guidelines for the diagnosis of comatose states as a result of findings indicating incorrect diagnoses adversely affecting care decisions.[30] A new proposal addresses the differentiation between a "persistent" vegetative state and a new category of "permanent" vegetative state.

The term *permanent vegetative state* suggests an irreversible condition in which there is a high probability that the person will not regain consciousness. This category would be applied to individuals who have been in a persistent vegetative state for twelve months after traumatic coma or for three months after non-traumatic coma[31] (although these time designations are still under debate). The use of this determination—or any other—is highly significant because it gives rise to a reevaluation of medical care, which may then lead to ethical and legal issues associated with potential withholding or withdrawal of life support equipment.

Brain Death

How to define death has been the subject of a very important discussion in recent times. Until the development of life support technology in the 1960s, comatose patients either improved or died quickly.[32] At that time, death was defined as the permanent cessation of the functioning of the heart and lungs. As a result of medical advancements, however, machines have made it possible to maintain heart and lung activities that, when previously left to their own levels, would otherwise have ceased. This prompted legislation in the 1970s in the United States to consider an alternative definition of death as the complete, irreversible loss of brainstem function. This determination must be confirmed by a second physician.[33] In the United States legal interpretations about the determination of death vary from state to state.

Any definition of death is highly significant because it has strong implications concerning the use or discontinuation of life support systems and the degree of medical care for comatose patients. Determining the presence or absence of death is one burden with which medical professionals and helpers must grapple repeatedly. Bear in mind that:

> …recuperative powers of the brain sometimes can seem astounding to the uninitiated, and individual patients whom uninformed physicians might give up for hopelessly brain damaged or dead sometimes make unexpectedly good recoveries. It's even more important to know when to fight for life than to be willing to diagnose death.[34]

The current definition of brain death increases the importance of learning to communicate with people in comatose states.

Ethical Questions

Thanatos ethics are ethical standpoints about death. In coma work we believe it is our ethical responsibility to attempt to consult not only family and medical staff about health care and life-and-death decisions about a comatose person, but also to make every attempt to ask the person in the coma.[35] Until recently, comatose patients were never consulted because we did not know how to communicate with them. Now that we know communication is often possible, consulting with people in comas becomes an ethical necessity.

When asked about life-and-death issues, most people want to go on living. Only rarely do we encounter people who say that they prefer to die. We usually want everyone to live, but that may not be the individual's wish. For example, a thirty-five-year-old woman with whom we worked told us through her communication that she did not want to live. We asked a number of times, two weeks in a row, and always received the same answer. We didn't want to believe it. She was only in her early thirties. Yet, each time she gave the same response. Her family decided to wait and not to take any medical action. Although life support was not removed, she did die shortly thereafter.

Documents known as "advance directives" such as the "living will" and "durable power of attorney for health care" can be drafted before a person becomes seriously ill and while the individual is competent and in an ordinary state of consciousness. These documents establish a legal basis for abiding by a person's choices relating to medical care if the individual were unable to give a "competent" opinion because of illness or injury, including appointing someone to act on the person's behalf in such an event. Typically, adults who sign living wills can state that if they were to fall into a comatose or vegetative state—and it was determined that death was imminent and life-sustaining procedures only delayed the inevitable—they request the removal of artificial life support.[36]

We need to realize that such important decisions made about life and death before falling into a coma arise from one state of consciousness—usually our ordinary state of consciousness. That is why it is equally important to consult comatose persons about their wishes when they are in a highly altered condition because, in such a current, altered state people sometimes have very different feelings and answers to questions about life and death.[37] It is difficult for any of us to imagine how we might actually feel were we to fall into a coma. Therefore information from both states is essential in the decision-making processes. We call this a *double-state ethics*.

In an article on recent controversies concerning assisted suicide in relation to the impending changes in a person's state of consciousness during Alzheimer's disease, Ellen Goodman notes the need for a double-state ethics: "Do I as a person of sound mind have the moral right to decide the fate of the person I would become? I may not want to live as that person but that person—my future self—may want to live."[38] In addition, decisions to limit or withhold medical treatment are often based on the assumption that the person no longer has a favorable quality of life. Yet, in their book on clinical ethics, Jonsen, Siegler, and Winslade state, "We usually do not know whether, and to what extent, these persons experience themselves as 'burdensome' to themselves or experience their life as 'of poor quality.'"[39]

Consulting someone in a coma requires learning special methods of communication, such as the use of yes-and-no questions that the person can answer.[40] A comprehensive ethical standpoint would include taking into account the person's prior wishes and the current wishes of family and the medical staff, as well as making every possible attempt to communicate with the comatose person about his wishes while in this altered state.

Pain Medication

Ethical considerations also arise when considering the use of pain medication such as morphine, which is given to minimize the pain of the comatose person. Even though pain medication clearly can be a most welcome relief, some dying people prefer the ability to communicate even when in intense pain. In this case the goal becomes maximum pain relief with minimum reduction of communication abilities and consciousness.[41] As we saw in Peter's case, pain medication can cloud the patient's access to consciousness and ability to communicate with those around him.

Pain relief is not only associated with physiologic relief, but also has spiritual, psychological, and social elements.[42] Indeed, sometimes when these forms of suffering are relieved, the experience of pain is lessened. Also, what appears as pain to us as outside observers may not, as we saw with Peter, be painful from the comatose person's inner perspective. Some of the expressions that look like pain may have different origins relating to the person's altered state. Again, learning to communicate with the comatose patient can help resolve fears and questions about pain. In any case, even when individuals are medicated, they are still there and available to their own awareness.

Summary of Learning from Chapter 2

❖ The definition of what constitutes a normal state of consciousness is determined by a given culture. In this state of consciousness the person is able to function reasonably well in everyday life.

❖ An altered state of consciousness is any alteration from this ordinary state of consciousness. Altered states span a wide range of experiences from the most mild form, such as momentary wandering of attention or feeling drowsy in the morning, to the most profound altered state of coma.

❖ All of us experience altered states throughout the day. They are the doorway to new aspects of ourselves, which lie outside our ordinary consciousness.

❖ Coma is the deepest altered state; in it, the person seemingly does not react to outer stimuli and is apparently unable to give feedback.

❖ As caretakers, we need to know about our own altered states in order to appreciate and relate to someone in a coma.

❖ Traditional definitions of coma in neurological journals are based on cause-and-effect factors, levels of consciousness that are present or absent, and prediction of outcome.

❖ Medical definitions of consciousness depend on the perceptions of an observer. An alternative approach is to elicit a description of consciousness based on the comatose person's inner experience. This method requires the ability to communicate with comatose persons in their altered state of consciousness and notice responses.

❖ Comas may occur as a result of structural brain injury, metabolic changes and near-death conditions, psychogenic factors, or a combination of these.

❖ Coma onset is often associated with increased pressure in the brain. Common causes of comatose states include alcoholism, stroke, and trauma. Coma can result from traumatic or non-traumatic injury.

❖ Generally, the deepest level of coma lasts from two to four weeks. If the person does not awaken from the coma, she enters into various degrees of semi-comatose states. These varying degrees of altered states also occur in people near death.

❖ Medical and behavioral tests are used to determine the origins and depth of coma, such as an EEG, CT or MRI and the Glasgow and Rancho Los Amigos scales.

❖ Brain death is a much debated issue. Given what we now know about communicating with people in comatose states, the development of double-state ethics requires an attempt to communicate with comatose people regarding their care, pain relief, and life-and-death matters.

Notes

1. These peak or spiritual experiences occurring during coma may have been patterned during the person's entire life, usually unknowingly. Arny has found that people's strong or chronic body experiences often mirror their earliest childhood dreams or memories. These are pictures of personal myths trying to come to realization in their lives.

   For example, Peter, the man mentioned in Chapter 1, became a very loving teacher just at the end of his life, which was patterned in his early experiences. His earliest childhood memory was of being with his two little sisters in bed on Sunday morning and having a very loving, happy time together. Now at the end of his life, he was getting back to that myth.

   I also remember a woman who dreamed as a child about being alone in a peaceful meditative state. At the end of her life, she was unable to move and began to teach others about the beauty of quietness and of meditating on each breath.

2. The foremost researcher on shamanism, Mircea Eliade, says that shamans enter a trance, leave the body, and ascend to the sky or the underworld to discover the source of a person's illness. (*Shamanism*, 5). Shamanic initiation is sometimes seen as a ritual death and resurrection (76). During a healing ceremony the shaman purposefully enters altered states to "contact and utilize an ordinarily hidden reality in order to acquire knowledge, power, and to help other persons" (Harner, *The Way of the Shaman*, 25). Sometimes the shaman is said to climb a tree to reach the sky in order to reach heaven. He or she transverses between the various states of consciousness, bridging ordinary reality with transpersonal realms (Nicholson, ed., *Shamanism*, 27).

3. See Arnold Mindell's *City Shadows* for more on the structure behind extreme states of consciousness.

4. Thanks to Dr. Ernie Stewart for this clarification.

5. Clayman, ed., *American Medical Association Encyclopedia of Medicine*, 294.

6. Ross, "A Comparison of the Medical/Nursing and Process Work Approaches to Coma," 24. Ross says the reticular activating system "is a network of neurons and tracts that extends from the lower brain stem into the pons, midbrain, thalamus and cerebral cortex. Any disruption to the R.A.S. will reduce the level of consciousness and lead to coma. The cerebral cortex controls the content of consciousness while the R.A.S. is the on/off switch."

   See Ross's article for more on emergency and long-term medical interventions for coma. Also, the Aitken Neuroscience Institute in New York has developed, for the first time in the history of neurosurgery, standardized "Guidelines for the Management of Severe Head Injury," which will help to improve emergency and ongoing treatment of head injuries.

7. Chuang, "Neuroradiological Findings in the Comatose Child," 73–81.

8. Plum and Posner, *The Diagnosis of Stupor and Coma*, 1–9.

9. For more on the minimally responsive state see Giacino et al., "Consumer Forum About Practice Guidelines for the Vegetative and Minimally Responsive States" (tape 43).

10. Plum and Posner, *The Diagnosis of Stupor and Coma*, 1. See also Fazekas and Alman, *Coma*, 3.

11. Victoria Hospice Society, *Hospice Resource Manual*, 11.

12. Multi-Society Task Force on the PVS, "Medical Aspects of PVS: Statement of the Multi-Society Task Force. Part I," 1501.

13. Young, Blume and Lynch, "Brain Death and the Persistent Vegetative State: Similarities and Contrasts," 388–393.

14. Ibid., 390.

15. Plum and Posner, *The Diagnosis of Stupor and Coma*, 3.

16. Andrews et al., "Misdiagnosis of the Vegetative State: Retrospective Study in a Rehabilitation Unit," 13–14.

17. From this perspective, the comatose person is not only a machine where the body and mind are separate. The comatose person is a living being. As yet, however, there are no statistics about this. Although many individuals will not be convinced that the potential for awareness is always possible, it would be premature to rule out this possibility until we learn more about altered states and communication.

   In *The Modern Shaman's Guide to the Universe*, Mindell states that "…anything like a complete description of consciousness involves descriptions from both the experiencer and the experimenter, from both the person in a personal state of consciousness and a doctor or physicist in the consensus reality of a given culture making repeatable measurements. Thus consciousness is a combination of experimentally verifiable observations and subjective experience in any given situation." In press.

18. Clayman, ed., *American Medical Association Encyclopedia of Medicine*, 201.

19. Gerri Haynes, hospice consultant, personal communication with the author, October 1996.

20. Plum and Posner, *The Diagnosis of Stupor and Coma*, 193.

21. Clayman, ed., *American Medical Association Encyclopedia of Medicine*, 294.

22. Conditions such as catatonia can also mimic comas. In such cases diagnosis is crucial, but can be quite difficult (Plum and Posner, *The Diagnosis of Stupor and Coma*, 305–311): "Determining the cause of coma or, at times, even whether an unresponsive patient suffers primarily from a physical or psychiatric illness can be challengingly difficult" (9). See Arnold Mindell's *City Shadows* for methods of working with catatonia and extreme states.

23. Hern, in *Vancouver Island Head Injury Society Newsletter*, 10.

24. Vancouver Island Head Injury Society, "Traumatic Head Injury."

25. From the New Jersey Head Injury Association (Edison, N.J.), quoted in Slater, with Kendricksen and Zoltan, *Coping With Head Injury*, 3. The Brain Injury Association (BIA) in its publication of basic information ("Basic Questions about Brain Injury and Disability") states, "For patients with moderate brain injury (surviving six hours or less of coma) over half will be able to return to school, jobs, and independent living within a year after injury."

26. Giacino et al., "Consumer Forum About Practice Guidelines for the Vegetative and Minimally Responsive States" (tape 43).

27. Clayman, ed., *American Medical Association Encyclopedia of Medicine*, 294.

28. Developed by Jennett and Teasdale. In Jennett, *Management of Head Injuries*, 77–93.

29. Hagen, Malkmus, and Durham, "Original Scale of Rancho Los Amigos Levels of Cognitive Functioning."

30. American Congress of Rehabilitation Medicine, "Recommendations for Use of Uniform Nomenclature Pertinent to Patients With Severe Alterations in Consciousness," 205–209; Andrews et al., "Misdiagnosis of the Vegetative State: Retrospective Study in a Rehabilitation Unit," 13–16.

31. Multi-Society Task Force on the PVS, "Medical Aspects of the Multi-Society Task Force. Part II," 1572. Also discussed in Giancino et al., "Consumer Forum About Practice Guidelines for the Vegetative and Minimally Responsive States" (tape 43). The term *persistent vegetative state* is used after someone has been in a coma for one month and includes the following criteria:

    No perception, either of oneself or the world.

    Periods of sleep and wakefulness alternating irregularly.

    The autonomic function of brain stem and hypothalamus are preserved.

    No indication of arbitrary reaction to visual, auditory, or tactile inputs.

    No indication that speaking to the person is understood or that the person is trying to speak.

    Missing control of urine function and defecation.

    Variably preserved spinal cord or brainstem reflexes.

    Thanks to Dr. Pierre Morin for this clarification.

32. President's Commission for the Study of Ethical Problems in Medicine and Biomedical and Behavioral Research, *Defining Death*, 21. This report continues: "If no other complication supervened and the patient did not improve, death followed from starvation and dehydration within days; pneumonia, apnea, or effects of the original disease typically brought on death even more quickly. Before such techniques as intravenous hydration, nasogastric feeding, bladder catheterization and respirators, no patient continued for long in deep coma" (21).

33. Clayman, ed., *American Medical Association Encyclopedia of Medicine*, 334; California Health and Safety Code, Section 7180 (1976), in Black, *Black's Law Dictionary*, 188.

34. Plum and Posner, *The Diagnosis of Stupor and Coma*, 314. See also Ross, "A Comparison of the Medical/Nursing and Process Work Approaches to Coma," for examples of people spontaneously recovering from seeming brain death.

35. Arnold Mindell, *Coma*, 97–102.

36. *The Columbia University College of Physicians and Surgeons Complete Home Medical Guide*, 54–55.

37. Jayne Garrison, in her article "Rushing Heaven's Door" (126), says that a sociologist at the Mayo Clinic found that because of aging or illness (not necessarily coma), people frequently change their minds about what constitutes a "tolerable quality of life."

38. "Choosing Life or Death for the Future Self," *International Herald Tribune*, March 8, 1996, 7.

39. Jonsen, Siegler, and Winslade, *Clinical Ethics*, 121–122.

40. See Arnold Mindell's *Coma*, Chapter 12. See Chapters 5 and 9 in this manual for an exercise on binary communication. Note: This form of communication, which requires developing communication with a comatose person through yes-and-no answers, is now widely known in medical circles, although it is not being used as a way of asking comatose persons their wishes. It is primarily used as a means of assessing the comatose person's ability to relate to those in ordinary consensus reality.

41. Jonsen, Sieger, and Winslade, *Clinical Ethics*, 131.

42. Ibid. See also Kearney, *Mortally Wounded*.

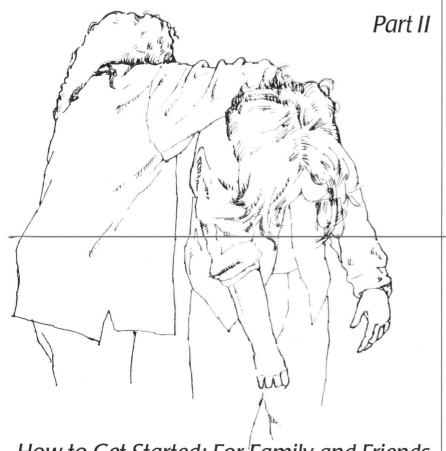

Part II

How to Get Started: For Family and Friends

W hen you as a family member, friend, or helper first learn that someone you love is in a coma, you need an overview of the situation. You need to know which medical and psychological questions to ask and what the answers mean. This chapter assists you in asking the central questions and gaining answers. Whether you are on site with the person or in another location connecting with the bedside situation by telephone, asking and getting answers to the following questions will help.

Ask the Following Questions

1. How did the person become comatose?

2. How long has the person been in the coma?

3. If there is structural damage as a result of oxygen deficiency, how long was the person without oxygen?

4. Were a CT scan, an EEG, an MRI, or other medical tests performed? What were the results of these tests?

5. What is the person's current health and medical condition? What is the view of the medical staff concerning the person's condition?

6. Does the comatose person have:
   - An oxygen mask or ventilator?
   - Intravenous tubes?
   - A tube inserted in the trachea to maintain the airway?

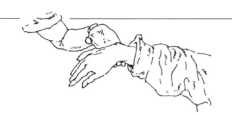

❖ Other medical equipment on which he is dependent?

❖ Special medications?

7. Is the comatose person receiving any rehabilitation treatments such as physical therapy?

8. How was the person's health before the coma?

9. If you don't already know it, find out something of the person's history, such as age, relationships, work situation, lifestyle, and education. Did the person ever speak about a childhood dream or childhood memory?

10. What was the mood of the person before she went into the coma? What was the last thing the person did or said before the coma? Did she have earlier periods of appearing absent, spacey, or depressed? Did she have previous comatose conditions?

11. What behaviors are observable at this time?

❖ What are the person's hands doing? Feet? Legs? Toes?

❖ What color is the face? Are there differences in color in different parts of the face?

❖ What position is the person sitting or lying in?

❖ What is the person's rate of breathing?

❖ Is the person making any movements?

  ❑ Are there spasms of the hands or feet?

  ❑ Is there decorticate posturing of the hands, in which the hands and fingers are rigidly bent in and upward toward the heart?

  ❑ Is there decerebrate posturing, whereby the arms are extended outward rigidly and turn away from the center of the body?[1]

  ❑ Are there any wild movements of limbs?

  ❑ If you pick up the arms, are they tense or flaccid?

❖ What are the person's eyes doing?

  ❑ Are they open?

  ❑ Do the pupils dilate?

  ❑ Do the eyes focus on anyone or anything?

  ❑ Do the eyes follow you if you move, or do they stay fixed?

12. Does the person give any noticeable response to communication from someone else?

   ❖ Have you noticed any responses to your communication?
   ❖ Have there been any responses that others are aware of? To whom or what?
   ❖ Does the person seem to make movements in response to what is happening in the room?
   ❖ Are there any responses that are repeated, such as finger movements, small eyebrow motions, or a slight turn of the head to the side?

13. Where is the comatose person?

   ❖ Is the person at home or in a medical facility?
   ❖ Is the family satisfied with the location? With treatment?

14. Does the person have a living will?

15. If you are a family member, how are you holding up? What is your mood? Are you depressed? If you are a caretaker, how are you feeling?

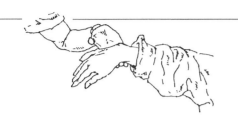

Discussion and Responses

1. The description of how the person became comatose will tell you whether the coma is due to structural damage or to metabolic changes near death, or is psychogenic. Knowledge of the type of coma will guide you when you attempt to communicate with the person. As mentioned previously, structural coma work involves basic coma methods, as well as special methods that follow the body's natural process of recuperation.

   Frequently, the greater the extent of brain damage, the farther away the signals of communication may be and the more difficult it can be to access them. Therefore it may take more time to feel that you are in contact with the comatose person. You can expect less or minimized feedback, and this work may require more time and patience. However, people do not operate like machines, and sometimes someone with more brain damage may recover more quickly and easily than someone with less. It is quite unpredictable.

   The person in a metabolic coma normally responds well to interventions and may achieve a degree of alertness and wakefulness in a short time. If the person is receiving morphine, however, responses may be delayed and require more time to appear. If the person becomes lucid, she may be able to tell you about her inner experiences.

   Psychogenic factors supporting the coma can be deduced by answers to question number 10. Methods for interacting with people in this type of coma are not different from those for coma of metabolic or structural origin.[2]

2. According to the Vancouver Island Head Injury Society "Even though improvements may continue over a lifetime, the most rapid recovery generally takes place in the first six months. This makes it very important for treatment to be received as quickly as possible to gain maximum recovery."[3] Plum and Posner state that the outcome is heavily dependent on the physician's proper emergency treatment even before a diagnosis is reached and in the very first hours after onset.[4] It is most helpful when you are also able to work with the person as

soon as possible following the onset of coma, once all medical interventions and emergency measures are complete. Most often, a younger person has a greater chance of coming out of a coma and of having less organic residual damage.

3. Generally, the greater the oxygen deficiency, the greater the amount of brain damage. When brain damage is extensive, feedback to your interventions may be delayed and you will need greater patience in your work. Structural brain injury requires the use of basic methods, as well as special coma methods (described in Chapters 6, 12, and 13).

4. The CT scan, EEG, and MRI indicate the extent and location of brain injury. Is the injury diffuse or local? Local injury refers to trauma that has occurred at a particular area of the brain and which can cause correspondingly specific defects in mental functioning, speech, or motor coordination, or paralysis.

5. Ascertain the current health and medical condition of the comatose person. Is the person near death or in the last stages of life? Is the person young and recuperating well? Has the person's chest been crushed? Does he have other injuries? Are there any other threatening medical conditions? This general health picture will give you an overview of the comatose person's overall condition and an awareness of particular physical conditions that you may need to be cautious and careful about.

6. If the person has an oxygen tube, ventilator, IV tubes, or other special equipment, she will not be able to move easily. You will need to be careful of this equipment during your work. Learn as much as you can from doctors and nurses about the medical technology, interventions, and medications being used. For example, some medications are used as sedatives, some to increase blood pressure, some to prevent seizures, others to remove fluid from the brain. Know that if someone is being given a lot of morphine, her response time may be delayed, as if dopey or drunk.

If you determine that the person is not in pain (by means of binary methods discussed in Chapters 5 and 9), you might consider, with the approval of medical and family, the possibility of lowering the amount of

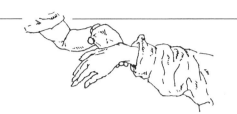

morphine or other painkillers, in order for the comatose person to gain greater access to her awareness and abilities to communicate with you.

7. Become informed about the kind of rehabilitation treatment the person may be receiving, such as physical therapy. Physical therapy is meant to decrease atrophy and help the body increase its strength and regain access to muscular coordination. Physical therapy follows a set program of methods for rehabilitation. In contrast, the methods in this book are geared toward following and responding to the spontaneous signals of the comatose person. These signals are part of the body's spontaneous method of communication and recuperation.

8. Gain an overview of the person's health before the coma. Was her health weak and failing, or was she strong and healthy? Did she have high blood pressure? Was she an overeater? Did she have high cholesterol levels? These may all be additional factors affecting the person's momentary condition. Also, if the person comes out of the coma and begins to reenter ordinary life, it will be important to consider any lifestyle changes that might influence her recuperation and overall health.

9. It is helpful to remember or know about the person's relationships, work situation, and lifestyle. However, when you work with the person in coma, avoid referring too much to this historical information. The person's state has changed, and he may not be relating to that history now. Again, this information will be of use to you if and when the person emerges from the comatose state and begins to adapt once again to everyday life.

   It is also helpful to know or remember whether the person ever mentioned a childhood dream or strong childhood memory. These dreams or memories are pictures of personal myths, which are often linked to strong body experiences such as coma. Knowing these mythic patterns may give you insight into the long-term, mythic experiences the person may be going through.[5]

10. Psychological factors such as depression, hopelessness about relationships, or prior times when the person seemed absent, forgetful, or distant may contribute to the comatose state. The last thing a person did or said before going into the coma may give you information about

background psychological issues related to the coma. It is important to know about these factors because if the person begins to return to everyday life, he may be confronted with these deep issues once again.

11. All of these observations will give you an overall idea of the comatose person's state and indicate doorways of communication. As discussed throughout Chapters 4-6 and 7-14, you can work with these signals by amplifying or deepening them through the use of movement, sound, or touch.

    Plum and Posner identify the indication of a light reflex in the pupils as "the single most important physical sign potentially distinguishing structural from metabolic coma."[6] In metabolic coma the pupillary reflexes are generally unaffected. In comas attributable to structural injury, however, the light reflex is disturbed. When a pupil is dilated, this can indicate that swelling of the brain is pressing the nerve to the pupil.[7] Sometimes the eyes remain open and become fixed or slowly rove. In coma work, all of these eye experiences are signals you should notice because, when you begin to work with the person, these signals can give you useful feedback.

12. Generally, the more response the better. No feedback may constitute negative feedback. Yet, if there is no response, that doesn't mean the person is incapable of doing so. She may need a rest, or those present may not be communicating with the comatose person in a way that is adapted to the person's altered state. Remember, too, that responses may be very minimal, yet extremely significant.

    Even if the person has a poor diagnosis and prognosis, if there is a great deal of feedback and response to your interactions, there is reason for hope and a good possibility for communication.

    Keep a log of signals and events that may be linked with feedback from the comatose person, such as a twitch of an eyelid when you come close or a strong response when the person's dog is brought into the room, when special music is played, when you touch the person's finger or hold her hand, when you pace the person's breathing, and the like. If you notice a consistent signal, you will be able to use that to develop communication in which the person can answer yes-or-no questions.

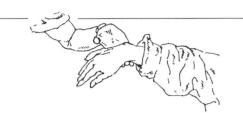

13. Of course, the family always wants to be sure their loved one is in a caring facility with well-trained medical staff. Frustration can be caused if family members believe that the facility is not suitable or feel that they are unable to communicate adequately with staff, or if moving the comatose person from one facility to the next has been required. As a coma helper, you can be of assistance and talk with the staff on behalf of friends or relatives.

14. If the comatose person has a living will, the family will most likely want to respect its directive, as well as take medical views into account. However, as noted in Chapter 2, it is also important to consult the comatose person about life-and-death issues now that he is in an altered state of consciousness (see Chapters 5 and 9 on binary communication).

15. As family and friends, talk about your feelings with the coma helpers. As a helper who is not necessarily part of the family, talk to family members about what is on their hearts and minds. Remember, such an experience is a terrible shock. The family may be under a tremendous amount of stress and need a great deal of support and time to talk to a caring, compassionate listener. Such experiences frequently evoke emotional and spiritual crises. Many family members, because of the high anxiety level of the situation, may stress themselves to the point of exhaustion. Family and friends should remember—and coma helpers should remind them—to take care of themselves, to not get sick themselves. The personal exercises in Chapter 7, especially Exercise 2, may be helpful.

Summary of Learning from Chapter 3

❖ Find out the origins of the coma. Is it due to structural damage, metabolic changes, psychogenic factors, or a combination of these?

❖ The most rapid recovery generally takes place in the first six months after onset of the coma. Therefore it is most important for the person to receive the earliest possible medical care and for coma workers to begin interacting with the person as soon as possible after all medical emergencies have been resolved.

- Generally, the greater the oxygen deficiency, the greater the amount of brain damage.
- The CT scan, EEG, and MRI help identify the location and extent of brain injury.
- Find out about the person's everyday life as background information for you. Do not stress this in your work because the person may not be relating to this information now that she is in an altered state.
- Psychogenic factors can affect comatose states. It is important to know these factors while working with the comatose person, particularly if the person begins to return to everyday life and must confront these issues once again.
- Obtain exact descriptions of the comatose person's behavior, body posture, signals, and movements to guide you in your work.
- Light reflex in the pupils is used in the medical context as a distinguishing factor between structural and metabolic comas.
- Learn to work with signals through movement, sound, and touch, as described in Chapters 4 through 12.
- If you, as a helper, or family members do not receive much response from the comatose person, it is possible that you are not relating to the comatose person in a way that connects to his present altered state or condition. It is also possible that the comatose person needs a rest.
- Keep clearly in your awareness all medical equipment that is in use as you work with the comatose person.
- Communicate with medical personnel about the kind of treatment being attempted, such as medication or physical therapy. If possible, if you are a helper, assist the relationship between medical staff and family when questions and problems arise.
- Family members should take time to talk about their feelings with the caregiver. As a caregiver, remember to listen to the feelings of family and friends.

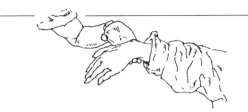

Notes

1. A technical definition of decorticate and decerebrate posturing: "Decorticate posture consists of internal rotation and adduction of the arms with flexion of the elbows, wrists and fingers… Extension of the legs may also be seen. Decerebrate posture may indicate more serious damage… The arms are stiffly extended, adducted and hyperpronated. There is also hyperextension of the leg with plantar flexion of the foot." (Lewis and Colliet, *Medical Surgical Nursing*, 1528-1529).

2. However, psychiatric conditions alone which mimic coma, such as catatonia, can be dealt with in other ways. See Arnold Mindell's *City Shadows* for methods.

3. Vancouver Island Head Injury Society, "Traumatic Head Injury." The Brain Injury Association (in "Basic Questions About Brain Injury and Disability") also says that rehabilitation for brain injury should begin as soon as possible, even when the person is in a coma.

4. Plum and Posner, *The Diagnosis of Stupor and Coma*, vii. See also "Coma" (program in the PBS *Nova* series).

5. See Arnold Mindell's *Coma* for more on myths and childhood dreams.

6. Plum and Posner, *The Diagnosis of Stupor and Coma*, 41.

7. "Coma" (program in the PBS *Nova* series).

Chapter 4

T his chapter and the next two give you skills and methods for accompanying a loved one in a comatose state, regardless of whether it is due to metabolic, structural, or psychogenic causes. This chapter and the next give the fundamental exercises that can be used for all types of comas. Based on the learning from this and the next chapter, Chapter 6 addresses the special needs of those in comas attributable to brain injury. The exercises in the following chapters build on one another.

Before starting, read over the following general points, which address fundamental qualities and practical tips for all aspects of coma work.

First Steps

❖ **Check on medical interventions.** The first step in coma work is to make sure all necessary medical interventions are as complete as possible before beginning your work.

❖ **Create relationship.** If you're a normal person you will be asking, "Why should I do all of these coma methods?" "Why should I touch 'Grandma' on the head, or notice her fingers moving, or get excited about a movement of her eyelid?" The answer is that the comatose person may experience your attempts at communication as an act of companionship and loving connectedness.

And, once the connection is created, you have the chance of unfolding her inner experience. Perhaps she will awaken—though

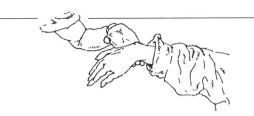

that's not the ultimate goal. Connection to inner experience is the goal. Loving contact, not separation. The person may begin to communicate with you or feel the support to go in another direction and follow her inner experiences.

❖ **Know that your feelings are an important tool**. Your effectiveness does not depend on your technique alone but on the feelings you have as you assist the comatose person. The techniques are one aspect of the work; your feeling sensitivity is the other. A loving, sensitive, and respectful contact with the comatose person is healing by itself.

❖ **Join the comatose person**. Coma work relies on your ability to communicate with the comatose person in ways that may be quite different from how you related to that person before her coma. Remember that the comatose person is in an extremely altered state of consciousness and you will need to adapt your communication style to this state. The methods will help you lessen the gap between your two realities. Although awkward and unfamiliar initially, with time these methods will become second nature.

One of the reasons our agony is increased when someone falls into a coma is that we feel we are not able to know where the person is or what she is experiencing. Coma work helps to relieve that feeling. Joining the comatose person in her communication style can heal some of the solitude and lack of intimacy connected with being in an isolated room or hospital. The comatose person is frequently relieved simply by being understood and joined in her inner experiences. For you, coma work relieves the loneliness of feeling out of contact with your loved one. Coma methods bring you into contact in a very deep and intimate way.

❖ **Do not press the person to relate to everyday reality.** Instead, join the person's experience by following his signals, for instance, by pacing the breath or commenting on small finger motions. In essence, you are saying, "I am here with you and I am going to join you where you are. You don't have to come out of your state in order to relate to me in 'ordinary' ways."

Coming out of a coma that was due to a brain injury from a car accident, one man wrote a poignant description of the frustration he felt when people disavowed his inner experiences. He wrote:

> ...I thought for some days that I was on an ocean liner with my wife, bound on a pleasure cruise... Or, I would imagine that I was on a desert island, surrounded by lapping waves.[1]

He continues:

> Gradually, as I became more oriented and more aware that "something had happened to me," the split between reality as seen by those around me, and as I interpreted it, became more painful. I would argue with those around me in defense of my fantasies.[1]

He is telling us that it is most important to understand a comatose person's experience from his perspective—that is, from the inside out.

❖ **Get physically close.** Get as physically close to your loved one as you can when using these methods. Before doing so, mention to the comatose person that you will be coming close to him. Then stand as close to the bed as possible or sit on the bed if conditions allow. Put your face close to the comatose person's ear when you begin to speak gently to him.

Being so close to your loved one may be very natural for you. However, if you feel uncomfortable, trust that the person in the coma appreciates your intimacy. Being in a hospital setting with very little physical or emotional contact can be isolating. Even a person who is ordinarily shy about contact appreciates close contact in a coma. We have never met a person who did not respond well to this kind of contact, when contact is made in a sensitive way. To perceive what this type of communication is like, it may be helpful to remember the intimate, sensitive way you have held, touched, or sung to a young child.[2]

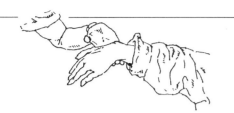

Exercises in Chapter 10 can help you explore your own shyness about touch and intimacy.

❖ **Mention what you will do before doing it**. Before you touch the comatose person, make sure you tell her what it is that you will be doing. If you are about to touch the person's wrist, say, "In a moment I am going to touch your wrist." Then wait a few seconds before doing so. The comatose person feels respected and can prepare inwardly for this contact. After some time, however, you will not have to mention everything you are doing.

❖ **Develop fluidity.** For learning purposes, I have developed individual exercises for many of the coma work methods. However, they are not really separate unto themselves. Once you have learned all the techniques, they will become a palette of tools you can call on depending on the comatose person's momentary signals and experiences. You will begin to communicate in a more fluid way, responding to the comatose person's momentary process rather than following a set of techniques.

❖ **Learn to communicate through signals.** All the movements, sounds, breathing patterns, changes in skin color, and muscular responses that you observe in the comatose person constitute the language of coma. These are the means through which the comatose person can communicate with you. If you notice these signals, the comatose person knows that you are aware of her communications. You will see these signals, hear them, or feel them with your hands. Even the most minimal signals from the comatose person, like a twitch of an eyelid, can be the doorway to communication. Coma methods will teach you to communicate in this language as well.

❖ **Amplify and unfold signals that you observe**. Amplification is a method in which you join the person in whatever inner experience he is having by following his signals and helping these experiences deepen and unfold through the use of sound, movement, breath, and touch. The exercises provide many different tools for amplifying various signals.

When you help the comatose person follow and unfold his experiences, sometimes this involves large-scale movements and sounds, and sometimes, very subtle, minute interactions. Know that very subtle, minimal, interventions which are related to the comatose person's inner state can connect deeply with him.

❖ **Follow feedback and timing.** One of your most important tools is the ability to notice the comatose person's feedback—her response to your communication. What you do depends on the feedback you receive. "Positive feedback" means that you get a response to what you are doing, for example, changes in breathing, changes in skin color, and movement. "Negative feedback" means the absence of any response. Know that responses may be delayed due to medication. Have patience, wait, and notice responses.

The frequency and duration of your work depend largely on the feedback you receive from the comatose person. If your loved one seems to be responding more and more, even if subtly, and you feel you are on track, stay with what you are doing and help that experience unfold. If you receive no feedback, however, take a break or try another method of communication (see Chapter 9 for more on this). When there is a lessening of feedback or the person seems to withdraw, that is a good time to take a break. You may also find yourself getting sleepy. This may be an indication that either you, or the comatose person, or both of you, needs a rest. Know that in coma work, doing less is better.

Keep in mind that, since the comatose person has been lying relatively immobile or without much physical exercise, any kind of physical exertion can be tiring. Make sure to watch the feedback. Stop what you are doing and take a break when the person seems to lose energy

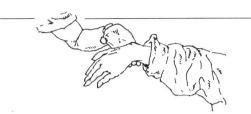

or interest. You will begin to receive less and less feedback from the comatose person and his attention will seem to draw away.

❖ **Notice your own trance states.** As some people interact with comatose people, they find themselves slipping into trancelike states in which dreamlike fantasies arise. This is quite natural, since you are aligning yourself with the altered state of the comatose person. Most of the time, it is beneficial to follow the signals of the comatose person. However, you might experiment with telling the person about your dreamlike images. Make sure to notice the feedback to your words. If you seem to receive a response, continue on this track. If not, try another method or take a rest.

For example, if you have a dreamlike image of the comatose person in a very peaceful state, floating on a river, you can tell the person your image. If the person does not seem to respond, return to mentioning the comatose person's actual signals. If you receive a response such as a big breath, continue speaking about the river, the sense of floating and peacefulness. Perhaps the person will react to one of these words strongly. Then continue to embellish verbally, saying something such as, "Hmm, so peaceful, not doing anything... just quiet... peace."

❖ **Use common sense and sensitivity.** As you interact with the comatose person, use your common sense. Don't disrupt the machinery connected to the person. Even the most gentle pressure on a person's chest when she has trouble breathing can be too much. Be very careful with any part of the body that has been injured. Don't pull on the joints of the leg if it has been injured, or press on tubes that supply food or oxygen! Also, make sure that you wash your hands before and after touching or working with the comatose person.

❖ **Discuss what you are going to do with other family members and friends.** If there are others in the room who don't know much about coma work, they may be shy about the ways you will communicate with the comatose person. Contact alone can make some people uncomfortable. So, first discuss what you are planning to do with other family members, and ask if your plan is permissible.

❖ **Practice with others.** If you have time, practice these techniques with a friend or family member. One of you should act as though you are in a coma, while the other practices the techniques. Then switch and try the other role. You will have a deeper sense of what it might be like to be in a coma and may even discover more about your own inner process. (You may want to try some of the exercises in Chapter 7 to assist you in exploring your own feelings about coma and altered states. You may also want to extend your learning by trying the intensive training methods in Chapters 8 though 13.)

❖ **Take care of yourself.** If a loved one is in a coma, it can be emotionally and physically distressing and tiring for you, and a terrible shock. The tension and stress alone can be very taxing on your own body. Don't forget to take care of yourself as much as possible.

Frequently Asked Questions

Can the comatose person hear me? Should I talk to her directly?

Always assume that the person in coma can hear you. Hearing seems to be the last faculty to deteriorate.[3] Speak to the person—don't talk as if the person is not there.

How many people should be in the room? Can we work together as a team?

It does not matter how many people are in the room. Try to involve the most sensitive people or those who may be standing shyly in the corner. (These people are often especially gifted in coma work.) It is helpful, although not imperative, that whoever is present be involved in what you are doing. If the others are willing, you can work as a team as described in

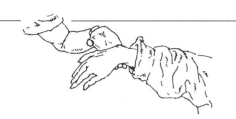

the exercises. Be aware that some of the exercises, particularly those related to structural coma, require more than one person.

What do I do if I see sadness or pain on the comatose person's face?

As you work with a loved one, you will notice, no doubt, many kinds of facial expressions. In coma, the use of muscles may be slowed or altered as a result of physical injury, or muscular expressions may originate from deep altered-state experiences. What looks like pain or sadness may be related to a kind of experience very different from those to which we are normally accustomed. Still, if you are worried that the person is expressing pain, you can use a binary form of communication to ask the person this question (see the exercise at the end of Chapter 5).

When you visit a comatose loved one, you naturally bring a lot of history with you. Keep in mind that the comatose person is in a very different state of consciousness than previously—most often quite unrelated to the way you have known him before. Try not to jump to conclusions or impose assumptions before getting feedback on whatever is concerning you from your loved one.

How can I explain what I am doing to medical or hospice staff?

Everyone involved in coma care is interested in the comatose person being as comfortable as possible. Although approaches may differ and time constraints are always limiting, most caretakers and health care professionals want to relate to the person in the most compassionate way. Methods enabling the comatose person to connect to her inner experiences and "speak" about them, or to answer questions, are of value to everyone. These methods relieve the frustration family members and medical staff alike have felt about not being able to intimately communicate with the person.

Exercises

As you begin each exercise, read through the entire instructions to acquaint yourself with the techniques. Then begin to apply the methods with the comatose person by following the abbreviated "Quick Review" that follows the instructions.

Exercise 1

Joining through the Breath

The first and most powerful way of contacting and joining the comatose person is to relate to her through the rate of her breathing. When you do this, the comatose person feels your presence. She feels accompanied and connected to. She has the sense that you are joining her inner experiences and pace of communication. The sensitive way you speak to and touch the person should, initially, mirror this breathing rate.

In this exercise, the person's breathing becomes the central guide for your interactions.

Instructions

1. **Enter, notice, and adjust.** As you enter the room, notice the position of the person's body on the bed, the general atmosphere in the room, and the pace of her breathing. Modify your own inner feelings so that they align more closely to this timing. Meditate with her and try to feel your way into her world. Tune in to the atmosphere. For example, if you are feeling a bit anxious, take some time to relax and enter into a slower pace. Use your intuition and feelings to sensitively enter into the comatose person's world.

2. **Get close.** Go as close to the bed as you can. Stand or sit comfortably.

3. **Put your head close and pace the person's breathing with sounds.** Slowly move closer. Put your head near the ear of the comatose person's head (Figure 1). Make soft exhaling and inhaling sounds that mirror the rate and strength of the person's breath.

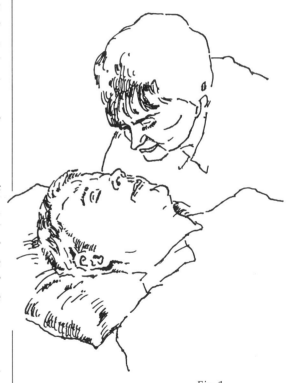

Fig. 1
Getting close and pacing the breath

4. **Speak in rhythm with the breathing rate.** In a loving, gentle voice, speak in the rhythm of the person's breathing. That is, speak when the person exhales, and pause during the inhale. Tell the person who you are and that you will be with her for a while. If your time is limited, it may ease you to say:

"I can be with you for [state the amount of time] this visit."

Here is an example of speaking in rhythm with the breathing:

[Comatose person inhales, and now on the exhale] "Hello, Alice. This is Amy. I'm here... [person inhales, and now on the exhale] I'm going to be with you for a while... [Person inhales, and now on the exhale] It's so nice to be here with you."

Suggest that the person trust her inner experiences. Say something like:

*"All you have to do *...is follow what is happening inside of you *...experiment with trusting in it *...whatever it is that you might be experiencing *...that will show us the way."*

Note: Asterisks (*) represent inhalation pauses.

5. **Touch and press the wrist.** After a few minutes, and in the rhythm of the breath and speaking on the exhalation, tell the person that, in a moment, you will touch his wrist. (We suggest touching the wrist because the wrist is far from the rest of the body; therefore touching it is a gentle, non-intrusive way to begin to make contact.)

Wait a few moments and then grasp the wrist (Figure 2). Gently press the wrist as the person inhales, releasing the pressure on the exhale. As an alternative, if the hand is on the stomach and it is more difficult or intimate to touch the wrist, do the same thing but with the elbow.

6. **Validate following inner experiences.** While pressing and releasing the wrist, continue to make sounds that mirror the rhythm and intensity of the person's breathing. Still in rhythm of the breath, say something like:

*"All you have to do *... is follow what is happening inside of you *... Experiment with trusting in it *... Whatever it is that you might be experiencing *...will show us the way."*

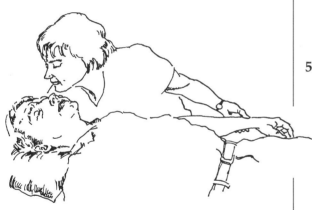

Fig. 2
Touching and pressing the wrist in conjunction with the breath

Notice responses to your communication such as deeper breaths. If you receive such positive feedback to pressing the wrist, remain there a while longer.

After a while you can try stroking the person's head or cheeks lovingly in rhythm with the breath. If you are comfortable, show the person some sign of affection—and tell her that you are there. If there are no injuries in the chest area, gently touch the bony part of the upper chest with the open, flat palm of your hand, pressing slightly as the person exhales and releasing this pressure on the inhale. In each case, continue to make comforting sounds that mirror the rhythm of the breath, and in this rhythm tell the person you are there and that she should try to follow her experiences.

The rule to remember is, if you get positive feedback such as a big breath, the head turning to the side, sounds, or small movements, even if they are quite small, stay with what you are doing. If you do not get much response to what you are doing, try adding new elements (suggested in step 7) slowly, piece by piece, joining the breath and watching for responses. If you receive a response, stay with what you are doing. If you don't get a response, try something new, relax, or take a break. Remember, in coma work, less is always better than more.

7. **Include others.** If there are others in the room, you can try some of the following suggestions.

Someone gently presses on the foot of the comatose person in rhythm with the breath. Tell the person:

*"John is here. He's going to go to your feet *... He'll hold them and gently press slightly."*

John then moves to the bottom of the bed and says, in rhythm with the person's breath:

*"This is John here at your feet *... I'm going to gently press your feet."*

John then gently presses up on the balls of the feet, gently flexing the foot as the comatose person inhales and letting go of the pressure on the exhale. Simultaneously, you continue with the wrist (Figure 3). Watch for feedback. If you receive responses, continue.

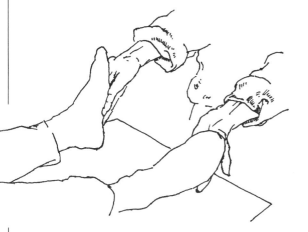

Fig. 3
Pressing the balls of the feet in conjunction with the breath

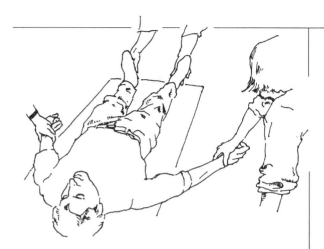

Fig. 4
*Pressing the other wrist in
conjunction with the breath*

Joining through the Breath

Quick Review

1. **Enter, notice and adjust.**
2. **Get close.**
3. **Put your head close, and pace the person's breathing with sounds.**
4. **Speak in rhythm with the breathing rate.**
5. **Touch and press the wrist.**
6. **Validate following inner experiences.**
7. **Include others.**
8. **Hum a tune.**

At another point you can add a third person to do the same thing with the other wrist in rhythm with the breath (Figure 4). As an alternative, two people, one on each side of the bed, can slightly lift each elbow and wrist as the person inhales, and gently let the arm down on the exhale. The person at the feet can now support and slowly lift the legs at the ankle in the same rhythm, and then let them down again.

Someone can also stand behind the person's head and, if the person does not have any complications or injuries there, gently press the crown on the inhalation and release on the exhalation with the palms of your hands.

As an alternative, cradle the head gently at the bottom of the skull where it meets the neck. Lift the head ever so slightly during inhalation, then slowly and gently let it down on the exhale (Figure 5). If you are working alone, you can move to these different parts depending on the feedback.

8. **Hum a tune.** Music seems to be one of the most basic elements of life; it is like an underground current, and most people seem to relate to it in a deep way. Using the kind of music the comatose person loves can forge a special link for him. If the person has a favorite song, hum or sing that song. Or hum a lullaby to the rhythm of the breath.

Do steps 1 through 8 for a few minutes, then take a break.

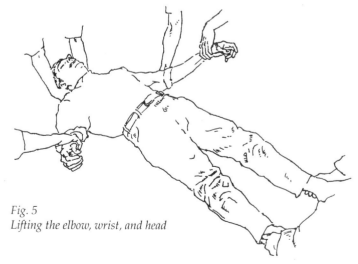

Fig. 5
Lifting the elbow, wrist, and head

Summary of Body Parts

Wrist	Press on the inhalation, relax on exhalation.
Chest	Gently press upper part of chest during inhalation, relax on exhalation.
Head and face	Gently stroke the head or face, or both, in rhythm with breath.
Feet	Press or flex balls of feet on inhalation, release on exhalation.
Other wrist	Press on inhalation, relax on exhalation.
Elbow and wrist	Lift during inhalation, lower during exhalation.
Leg	Lift at ankle on inhalation, let down on exhalation.
Crown of head	Gently press crown on inhalation, release on exhalation.
Bottom of skull	Lift slightly on inhalation, lower gently on exhalation.

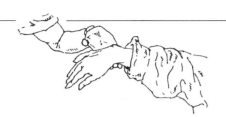

Exercise 2

Sensory-Oriented Coma Work

Sensory-oriented refers to the way we experience ourselves through our senses, that is, through seeing, hearing, feeling, smelling, or moving. The comatose person may be experiencing visual images, hearing or making sounds, having inner feelings, or making physical motions. These are the most common sensory experiences we see in practice. Smell is also a sensory channel, although we won't be focusing on it much in this manual.

Suggesting various sensory modes and noticing responses allow us to get in contact with the comatose person and help that person focus on and unfold his inner experiences.

First, we repeat earlier methods, then add the sensory work. If you do not detect a response, simply encourage the person to follow his inner world.

Instructions

1. **Get close, pace breathing, and press the person's wrist.** Come into the room, notice the person's rate of breathing, and adjust yourself to this rhythm. Sit close, say you are there, and gently press the wrist when the person inhales. Speak in the rhythm of the breath.

2. **Talk about following inner experience.** Pacing the breath, say something like:

   *"All you have to do *… is follow what is happening inside of you *… experiment with trusting in it *… whatever it is that you might be experiencing *… This will show us the way."*

3. **Mention sensory channels and respond to feedback.** As you pace the rhythm of the comatose person's breath, say:

   *"You might be **feeling** things *… or you might be **seeing** things *… or **hearing** things * … or making **movements** *… If you are **feeling** something then feel it; (pause briefly for a reaction)* … if you are **seeing** something, then look at it; (pause as above) *… if you are **hearing** something, then listen (pause) *… ; if you are **moving**, then follow these movements (pause)."*

Watch for feedback as you mention these different channels, and encourage the person to continue in whichever channel there is a response. For example, if the person takes a big breath in response to one sensory channel, then speak more about that channel. Let's say the person takes a deep breath when you mention *seeing*. This could be encouraged by talking about seeing or vision in a general way, without specific content. For example:

"Oh, seeing... yes, I see that, too... amazing, looking... Yes, seeing, look, watch...."

Here are some examples connected with other sensory channels:

"Listening, hmmm, sounds, hearing, just listen..."

"Feeling, yes, sensations, feel what you are feeling..."

"Yes, little movements, hmmm, moving...."

If you are unsure about which channel the person experiences himself in, just encourage the person in a general way to follow whatever he is seeing, hearing, or feeling, or any small movements that arise.

4. **Stay with the area where you get the most feedback.** Notice where you get the most response, and continue to encourage the person there. If the person seems to be looking at something, continue to talk about seeing. If he is hearing something, encourage him to continue to listen closely, and so on. Continue to encourage the person to follow his awareness of whatever is happening.

Once you have tried this sensory coma work, continue with Exercise 3, which helps you learn to respond more fully to signals from the comatose person.

Sensory-Oriented Coma Work

Quick Review

1. **Get close, pace breathing, and press the person's wrist.**
2. **Talk about following inner experience.**
3. **Mention sensory channels and respond to feedback.**
4. **Stay with the area where you get the most feedback.**

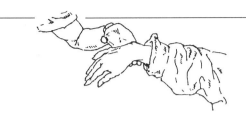

Exercise 3

Sensitive Communication and Responding to Signals

You may have noticed that the comatose person makes subtle signals, such as slight movements, sounds, gestures, or twitches. Some of these may be quite small, but are, nevertheless, very significant. Attending to even the most minimal signals is very important; they are the beginning of communication and indicate the presence of inner experiences.

When you notice these signals, the comatose person will feel accompanied and know that you are aware of her communications. Also, you help the comatose person, first, become aware of her process; second, gain the ability to follow and complete inner experiences; and, third, have the possibility of using these signals to communicate with you if she so desires.

Instructions

1. **Notice signals.** Watch for very tiny signals, such as the slight raising of an eyebrow, twitching of the face, movements of the mouth, swallowing, movements of the limbs, motions of the fingers, deeper or shallower breaths, slight head movements, various kinds of sounds, changes of color in the face, opening of the eyes, or turning of the head. You may also notice more apparent signals, such as thrashing in the bed, head jerking to the side, or sudden, loud sounds.

2. **Respond to each signal.** Whenever you observe one of these signals, let the person know that you notice it. All of us know how comforting it is to be attended to— for someone to notice, in a caring way, the very small signals that we make.

   Every time the person makes a signal, comment with an interested, excited tone. For example, if you notice an eyebrow move, you might say, *"Oh, that eyebrow!"* When you comment on particular signals, however, try not to add any interpretative comments. Simply remark on exactly what you are seeing. We call this *blank accessing*, in which you let the comatose person know in words or affirmative sounds that you have noticed a particular signal. Here are some examples of methods of response:

"Sometimes your head moves on its own, just like that."

"Yes, those lips move, I see them."

"Wow, a big breath, that's important."

"Oh, yes, I see that you can move your finger."

"I saw that shrug."

"I saw your eyes flicker a bit and your eyebrow move. Yes, that's very important to me."

"Amazing to see your mouth move, yes... you are saying something."

"Oh, your mouth is moving and your leg is moving!"

"Mmmm, I like the way you use your fingers. Yes, I feel them squeezing my hand. Wow! I know you're there. You can squeeze my hand to communicate with me."

"Oooh, that sound, what an amazing sound. I heard it."

If you are not quite sure what is happening, you can also make general statements, such as:

"Oh, you are experiencing that!"

"Oh, I didn't realize that!"

"Little movements are interesting— yes, moving!"

"Go ahead and follow your movements now, even if you don't know where they are going."

Or simply make affirmative sounds when you notice a signal, such as:

"Uh-huh, oh, yeah, mmm, that's right."

"Mmm, wow!"

3. **Gently touch the body part that is moving.** If you see the mouth move, you can touch it gently and say:

"Wonderful to see your mouth move" (Figure 6).

If the person's head moves slowly to one side, gently put your hands on the head and encourage him to continue with that motion.

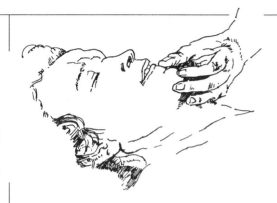

Fig. 6
Touching the mouth

A note about interpretation: People appreciate your interest in their signals, even if you do not always understand the message correctly. All of us have a tendency to interpret what we are seeing and imagine what the comatose person might be experiencing. We think particular signals mean this or that. For example, we think that when someone's brow is scrunched, the person is worried. Frequently, however, these ordinary interpretations are *not correct* when that person is in a coma. The inner experiences people are having during altered states are often quite different from what we imagine from our perspectives in everyday reality.

If you do have an intuition about the person's experience, try saying it, and notice the response. If the person seems to respond even more to what you are saying, continue. Elaborate on the words or feeling that the person seems to be responding to (see the short example in Chapter 11, exercise 3, step 7). If you interpret a particular signal in the wrong way, however, it will probably not disturb the person too much. She will simply retreat more and give less feedback.

If the person does not respond to your intuitions, return to simply mentioning the signals you see without adding much content. The important element is noticing the feedback. If you get a positive response to what you are saying, continue in that direction (see the example of feedback in Chapter 7).

4. **Match your responses to the signals.** When the quality of your response mirrors the quality of the signal, it helps the person become aware of what he is doing. Through sounds and words, mirror the quality, strength, and rhythm of the signal you are noticing. For example, when you hear a sound, make a similar sound in return. A slow, gentle turn of the head to the side could be mirrored by a slow, gentle, drawn-out sound, starting when the movement begins and ending when the movement stops. A more dramatic, accented movement should be followed by a sound or word that mirrors the intensity and staccato nature of the movement expressed. A slight flick of a finger might be followed by a short *"Yeah!"* Using sounds to communicate is a very direct and natural way of interacting.

5. **Notice the person's responses, and interact.** Notice whether you gain any responses from the comatose person when you mention certain signals. For example, you might notice that the upper lip twitches. You mention this, and then the lip twitches again. This is a response. You can then interact with the person by saying:

   "Oh, yes, I see that… you can move your lips… Wonderful lips!… Go ahead and move them… I notice them… yes… I know you're here when you do that."

   Continue to communicate sensitively with this signal by focusing on it, using more blank-access statements, touching the lips gently with your fingers, and encouraging the person to follow his experiences. Later, he may be able to use that lip motion to communicate with you (see the exercise on binary communication in Chapter 5).

   If you tell the comatose person that you notice her fingers moving and then her fingers grasp your hand, you might say:

   "Oh, I know you are here when you squeeze my hand. Yes, I feel you, how wonderful to feel you here."

6. **Add sound, and develop additional communication.** Once you begin to make sounds with someone, you can start a communication system by adding more sounds. We all remember this basic way of

communicating with a child by repeating sounds they make and starting a "conversation" in this way.

If the comatose person says "*ahhh*" you can also say "*ahhh*." Make sure to use the same intensity, volume, and energetic feeling in your sound as hers. Now try to add sounds. After a while, try a different inflection or rhythm to your sounds (such as "*ahhhh-ah-AH!*"), and notice what kind of feedback you get. If you do not get any feedback, try adding a slightly different combination of sounds or intonation, for example, "*ahhh, ah, WHOOO-woah!*" If the comatose person responds with more sounds, then you know that you have laid the foundation of a whole new communication system.

Note: Although most of us think we should be quiet when someone is in a coma, it is more helpful to match our sounds to the intensity and quality of the comatose person's expressions. If the person has a lot of intensity in what she is doing, she will feel related to if you join her rhythm and quality of expression. (For an example of many of the above coma work methods, and to gain a sense of the flow of the work, see the examples after Exercise 8 in Chapter 8.)

Sensitive Communication and Responding to Signals

Quick Review

Begin with the steps in exercise 1, "Joining Through the Breath." Then continue as follows:

1. **Notice signals.**
2. **Respond to each signal.**
3. **Gently touch the body part that is moving.**
4. **Match your responses to the signals.**
5. **Notice the person's responses, and interact.**
6. **Add sound, and develop additional communication.**

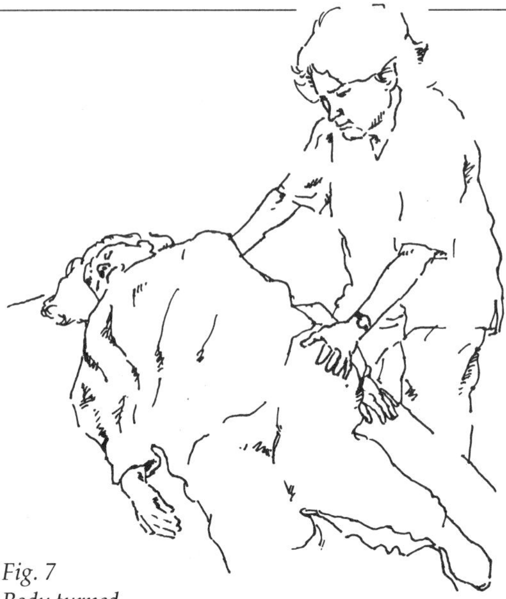

Fig. 7
Body turned
partly to the side

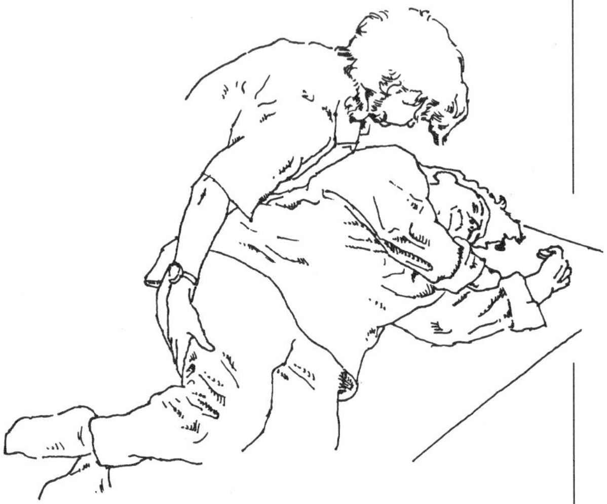

Exercise 4

Noticing Posture and Position

Among the strongest signals you notice from the comatose person are her overall posture and the position of body parts: the general posture of the body, the direction the head is facing, the way the hair has fallen, the position of the hands, the placement of the legs. Connecting with these signals, again, gives the comatose person the sense that you are in loving contact with her.

In this exercise you assist the person's body and postural expressions by encouraging these signals with your hands. Your touch helps the comatose person gain access to any experiences that are expressed through her body posture. Remember to continue to make affirmative sounds acknowledging and accompanying the person's signals.

Fig. 8
Encouraging body posture
toward the side

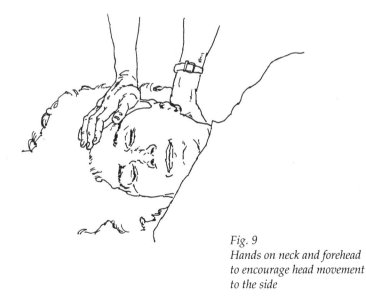

Fig. 9
Hands on neck and forehead
to encourage head movement
to the side

Instructions

1. **As before, pace the comatose person's breathing and notice signals.**

2. **Notice body posture and position, and use your hands to encourage.** Following are some possible body signals you may encounter and methods of encouraging them. Again, remember to mention verbally what you are going to do before doing it.

   ❖ If the body is turned partially to the side, gently curve the person over a bit more in that direction by using your hands on her back. Sometimes people curl up in a fetal position. Touch or stroke the person on the back in a caring way (Figures 7 and 8). Gentle and soothing sounds are helpful here.

   ❖ If the head is slightly turned or leaning to one side, use your hands to gently move the head just a bit further in that direction: place your hand on the person's cheek and gently press. Or place your hands behind the neck and back of the head, and gently help the neck muscles and head turn in that direction. Stroke the head in the direction it is facing (Figure 9). If you do this, it is possible that the person may turn her head even more toward you. Or, if the person's head starts to rise, place your hands behind the upper back, neck, and head to assist the movements (Figure 10).

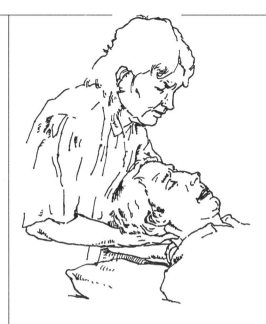

Fig. 10
Assisting the head as it rises up

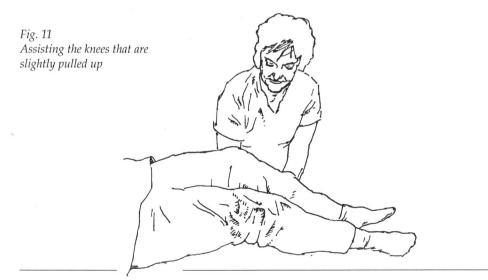

Fig. 11
Assisting the knees that are slightly pulled up

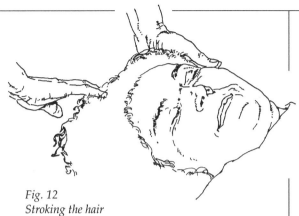

Fig. 12
Stroking the hair

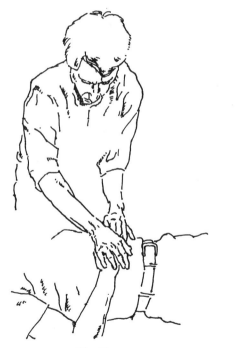

Fig. 13
Putting hands gently
on the person's hands

❖ If the person is lying on her back and her legs are pulled up slightly at the knees, support the knees from underneath and draw the legs up a bit further (Figure 11).

❖ Similarly, notice the direction in which the hair is combed or has fallen. Gently stroke the hair and head in that direction (Figure 12).

❖ Notice where the person's hands are, and gently rest your hands on top of them. For example, if the person's hands are on her stomach, place one of your hands on top. This may bring warmth and awareness to the stomach area (Figure 13). Or, if one hand begins to rise slightly, put your fingers under the wrist or elbow, and through gentle, supportive touch, encourage the person to follow this movement (Figure 14).

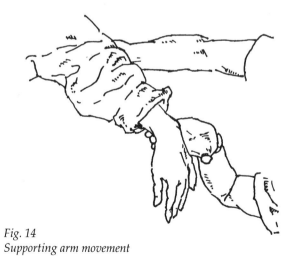

Fig. 14
Supporting arm movement

- ❖ If breathing is the strongest signal, after establishing contact—and if there are no complications in the chest area—place your hand lightly on the person's upper chest. Press very gently as the person exhales, and release on the inhale (Figure 15).
3. **Notice signals and respond.** Notice any responses you receive, and continue to remark about and sensitively interact with them.

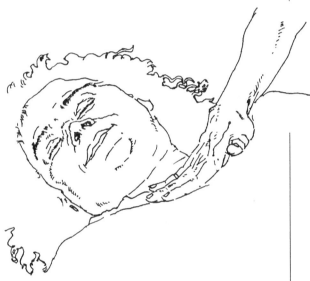

Fig. 15
Gently pressing on upper chest

Noticing Posture and Position

Quick Review

1. **Pace the comatose person's breathing, and notice any signals.**
2. **Notice body posture and position, and use your hands to encourage.**
3. **Notice signals and respond.**

Summary of Postures and Positions

Body turned partially to side	Gently move it in that direction.
Head turned or leaning to one side	Gently move it in that direction. Gently press or stroke cheek in same direction. Put your hands behind the neck and head, and gently turn them in same direction.
Head begins to rise up	Place your hands behind the back, neck, and head, and assist the movement.
Knees raised up slightly	Support from underneath the knees and ankles, and draw the legs up a bit.
Hair	Stroke in direction it is combed or has fallen.
Hand position	Gently rest your hands on top of them.
Hand rises slightly	Put your fingers under the wrist and elbow, and support the hand.
Breathing	Press gently on the upper chest on exhalation, release on inhalation.

Summary of Learning from Chapter 4

❖ Get physically close to the comatose person, and use your feelings and sensitivity to join him.

❖ Join the person's rate of breathing by speaking and touching in rhythm with the inhalations and exhalations. Speak on the exhale.

❖ Talk to the person, knowing that she can hear you. Suggest that she follow her inner experiences.

❖ Mention the various sensory channels and notice any responses.

❖ Don't interpret. Simply respond to the kinds of signals you observe, and match your responses to their quality and tempo. If you do decide to express an intuition, watch the feedback and adjust.

❖ Notice any responses, and add sound to develop additional communication. Make sure your sounds and words match the quality and rhythm of the comatose person's signals.

❖ Notice overall body posture and position. Increase the person's sense of her body and its postural expression by encouraging these signals with your hands.

Notes

1. See Frederick R. Linge's article "What Does It Feel Like to Be Brain Damaged?" which gives an excellent description of the experiences of brain damage.
2. Thanks to Debbie Hart for suggesting this.
3. Kay Ross, RN, Coma Work Theory and Training Class, Process Work Center of Portland, Oregon, Fall 1995.

he exercises in this chapter deepen those described in Chapter 4. The methods involve following the comatose person's inner experiences by:

1. Using movement to access experiences in various parts of the body.

2. Using your hands to discover experiences in the face.

3. Developing a method of asking questions and gaining answers.

Exercise 1

Moving the Body

The next step in your coma work is to gain access to any experiences the person may be having in his hands, arms, legs, or head. In the exercises in Chapter 4, you touched or moved these parts in response to signals. In this exercise, you are exploring these body parts to see if a response awaits you. Your touch helps bring awareness to, and facilitates the expression of, the person's inner experiences. It helps the comatose person become aware of his movement tendencies and express himself more fully through them.

The idea behind all this is to knock on the doors of the unknown, to release and discover what may lie in the depths of the comatose person. Therefore, move the body slowly and sensitively by lifting parts of it, millimeter by millimeter, and noticing any responses in the muscles or tissues. Then encourage the comatose person to focus on and follow these responses. In essence you are relating to the potential significance

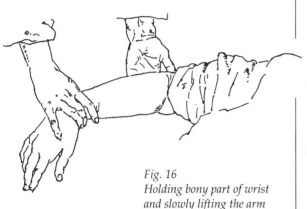

Fig. 16
Holding bony part of wrist
and slowly lifting the arm

of such movements and gestures and helping these experiences, which may be in the midst of expression, complete themselves.

If the person has been injured in any of these body parts, be very careful or do not move the part at all. Check with the medical staff if you are unsure.

Instructions

Begin with Exercises 1 and 2 in Chapter 4 and then continue.

1. **Tell the person you are going to lift the arm.** Tell the person that, in a moment, you will lift his arm. Then gently take hold of the bony part of one of the person's wrists with your hand.

2. **Move the arm gently.** Place the fingers of your other hand under the person's elbow to support the weight of the arm. Slowly and sensitively begin to lift the arm slightly upward and outward, millimeter by millimeter, bending the arm slightly at the elbow (Figure 16).

3. **Notice physical responses with your hands.** Continue to move the arm up and slightly side to side. As you do this, notice any feedback you receive. Some feedback is very subtle. For example, you may sense slight shifts, twitches, or tensions with your fingers. Other feedback involves larger muscular or tissue responses, such as flaccidity in the arm, resistance, tension, heaviness, changes in temperature, shaking, spontaneous motions, or the arm remaining suspended in the air. Encourage the person to follow these experiences.

It is very hard to describe muscular feedback. Discerning the varying kinds of muscular feedback requires a sensitive touch that develops over time. As you move parts of the body, your hands are like antennae that notice even the slightest responses, including movement and temperature changes.

4. **Experiment with strengthening the feedback.** Amplify responses by encouraging the person to follow the experience in her arm. You can amplify or deepen movement processes in a number of ways. Here are some suggestions:

❖ Follow the direction of the movement. If the arm is moving slightly to the right, you can use your hands gently to reinforce this movement and direction to the right.

❖ Resist the motion. You can slightly resist the direction of the movement. If the arm is moving to the right, give gentle resistance to the left (Figure 17). Slight resistance often helps the person get in touch more strongly with the impulse behind what she is doing.

❖ Use affirmative sounds and words to encourage the person's movements and experiences. Always use sounds and words that mirror the strength and quality of the movement. If there is a lot of tension, use straining and energetic sounds. If the arm is relaxed, use gentle, soothing sounds. If you notice something happening but do not know exactly what it is or how to mirror it, simply say:
"Oh, I felt a little something, go ahead, just follow it!"

❖ If you lift a body part and it freezes in place, encourage the person to visualize what she is doing. Say:
"Yes, looking, seeing, watching…"

❖ Amplify the sense of limpness or tension. Two of the most common muscular responses you will notice at varying times are flaccidity or tension. A relaxed, flaccid tone can be amplified or deepened by using soothing, gentle, massage-like contact. Tension can be met with an action of increased strength such as resistance. See later discussion for examples.

5. **Amplify any responses throughout the body.** Following are some ideas for assisting and amplifying these experiences throughout the person's whole body.[2]

❖ Relaxed: The arm may be very heavy and flaccid, and drop down loosely. This most often signals an internal, vacation-like experience, where the person is feeling relaxed and letting go of tension. If this appears to be the case, you can use any of the following techniques to help the person experience this throughout her body, always watching for feedback.

    ▫ Stroke or touch different parts of the body in comforting, soothing movements.

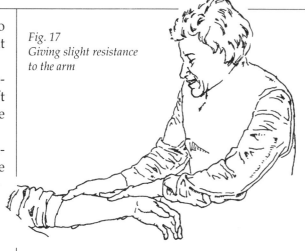
Fig. 17
Giving slight resistance to the arm

Note: The medical view of tension in the form of movements, gestures, or postures is to reduce the tension as soon as possible. According to this view, the body basically functions as a machine without an intelligence of its own. Although this viewpoint has value in certain areas, it is insufficient when we consider working with comatose people whose only means of communicating are through the subtle—and intelligent—signals given by their bodies.[1] Tension, while medically viewed as unwanted spasms, when unfolded, often indicates that a lot of energy, and perhaps a struggle, is occurring. When this energy is allowed to express itself, the spasms and tension frequently dissipate and are relieved. Flaccidity in the limbs usually indicates a sense of relaxation.

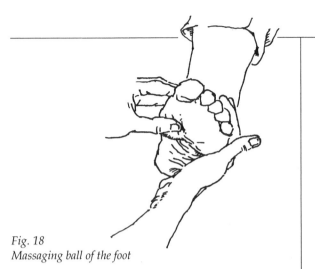

Fig. 18
Massaging ball of the foot

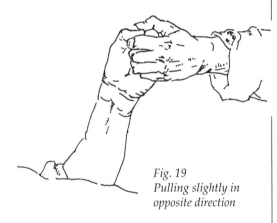

Fig. 19
Pulling slightly in opposite direction

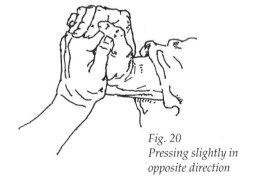

Fig. 20
Pressing slightly in opposite direction

- Gently massage the body.
- Cup the palms of your hands, and put your palms on the top of the head. Press very lightly as the person exhales, and relax as the person inhales.
- Stroke the head.
- Massage the balls of the feet, between the big toe and next toe, but not on the bone (Figure 18).
- Put your hands behind the person's back, especially when the person is sitting up, and massage the area gently.
- Talk in a low, soft voice that goes along with this relaxed state. Make soothing sounds. Children's songs are good during these times.
- Speak about relaxing things, saying such words as:

  "You're on vacation, going far away. You don't have to do anything. Down at the bottom of the sea… Enjoy it, I like being with you… letting go, you're a teacher of relaxation."

❖ Tensed: If the arm is tense or stiff, or pulls away from you, the person is most often involved in a wakeful, energetic process. Stiff and spastic movements often carry experiences of strength and, possibly, inner conflict or self-empowerment. These are subtle differences you can only feel with your fingers. If there is tension:

  - Match the person's energetic state by making more intense, louder, encouraging sounds or words like:

    "Whooah! Great! Wow, you are strong! Yes, I feel you, you're all here! Strength!"

  - Test and gently pull in the opposite direction of the tension while encouraging the person to pull away from you and use her strength (Figure 19).
  - If the person's hand and arm are stiff and pushing outward, press slightly in the opposite direction (Figure 20).
  - As you do this, notice any feedback. If the person seems to interact more with you, then you are on the right track. If not, stop and try another method or take a break. (See the discussion

in Chapter 8, page 160, for more on feedback.) If the person's hand and arm are pulling inward, pull outward slightly in the opposite direction.

- ☐ Press slightly on the balls of the feet, and notice whether the person pushes back. If so, give a bit more resistance while encouraging him to use his strength to push back at you (Figure 21).

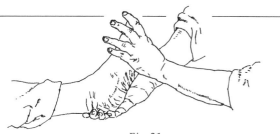

Fig. 21
Pressing slightly on balls of feet

- ❖ There may be many more responses. If so, try to amplify them slightly in other parts of the body. For example, if the person's arm is shaking or wobbling, you can gently wobble his knees or feet or other arm.

Be sure to watch the person for signs that he is becoming tired, and take a break then, encouraging the person to relax.

6. **Notice other signals.** At the same time, notice any other signals the comatose person is making, and use all skills learned until this point.

7. **Try steps 1 through 6 with the feet, a hand, a leg, the head, or a shoulder.** If you do not seem to gain much response from moving the arm, take a break or try the following. Tell the person that you are going to slowly lift the leg (or hand, shoulder, or head). Remember, it is always best, in the beginning, to tell the person what you are going to do just before you do it.

When you (or the other person) make contact with that body part, say:

"This is Amy here at your feet [or other body part] and I'm going to slowly lift your leg [or other body part]."

Additional suggestions for working with a leg, a hand, a shoulder, or the head include the following:

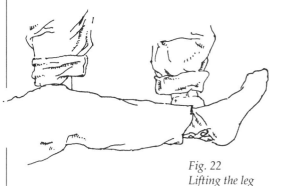

Fig. 22
Lifting the leg

- ❖ Lift the leg. When you lift the leg, support it under both the knee and ankle. Gently move the leg up and outward, bending it slightly at the knee. Slowly move the leg up and down and side to side, and notice any subtle feedback that you receive (Figure 22).
- ❖ Work with a hand. Place your hands in the person's hand and slowly stretch out the fingers. You will notice whether the fingers are flaccid (Figure 23) or cramped (Figure 24). Follow and respond to any feedback.

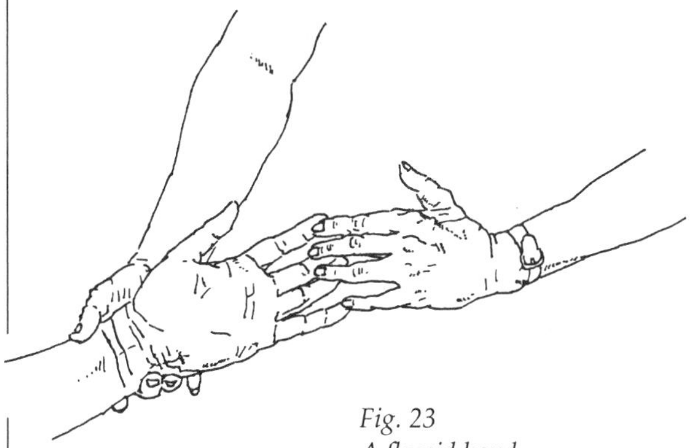

Fig. 23
A flaccid hand

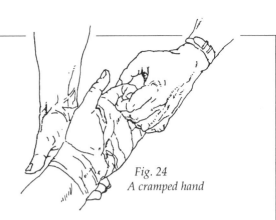

Fig. 24
A cramped hand

The hands and arms of many people with brain injuries are often bent inward and upward toward the heart (Figure 25) in a gesture known as "decorticate posturing." Or, one or both hands are turned away from the core of body and upward (Figure 26) in a gesture called "decerebrate posturing." In either case you can try to gently pull the thumb and fingers outward, and notice what happens in response. The fingers may be tense and retract even more. If so, slightly increase your pull, and encourage the comatose person to follow the strength of retraction in his hands (Figure 27). You may also pull gently on the wrist and notice responses.

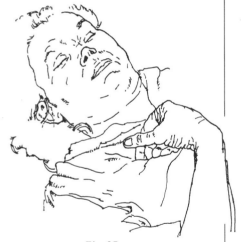

Fig. 25
Decorticate posturing

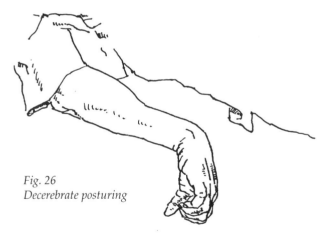

Fig. 26
Decerebrate posturing

❖ Lift the head. Support the head with the cupped palms of your hands at the base of the skull. Gently and very carefully, lift the head and move it minimally from left to right, up and down, and rotationally on its axis at the base of the skull. Notice any feedback (Figures 28 and 29).

If the head begins to turn slightly to one side, you can follow the direction of the movement with your hands in a loving way. Stroke the person's hair, and encourage him to move his head in that direction, or run your hands gently on the scalp in the opposite direction from the way the head is turned. In any case, encourage the person verbally by telling him that the head is moving beautifully in the right direction.

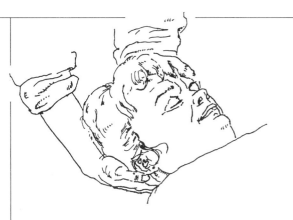

Fig. 28
Lifting head and moving it side to side

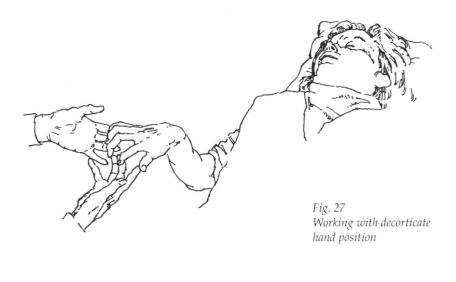

Fig. 27
Working with decorticate hand position

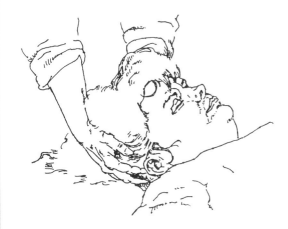

Fig. 29
Rocking head back and forth on its axis

Note: As you begin to connect with the comatose person, you will no longer need to mention everything that you are going to do ahead of time. Your relationship and work become more intimate and fluid. You will also be able to stop following the person's breathing rate exactly and simply continue to sensitively interact.

❖ Test the shoulder area. Place one hand underneath the shoulder blade and another on the upper chest. Gently draw the shoulder outward, and notice any responses (Figure 30).

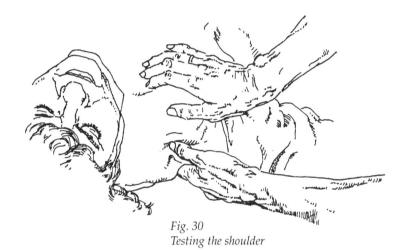

Fig. 30
Testing the shoulder

Moving the Body

Quick Review

1. **Tell the person you will lift the arm.**
2. **Move the arm gently.**
3. **Notice physical responses with your hands.**
4. **Experiment with strengthening the feedback.**
5. **Amplify any responses throughout the body.**
6. **Notice other signals.**
7. **Try steps 1 through 6 with the feet, a hand, a leg, a shoulder, and the head.**

Exercise 2

Working with the Face

Again, your hands are very important tools in coma work. By using your hands in a sensitive way, you bring awareness to the comatose person's internal experiences. Areas of the face such as the eyes and mouth are some of the most basic communication centers from which we experience and express ourselves.

Although neurologists view various kinds of responses such as yawning, grimaces, or decorticate posturing as automatic, "primitive" reflexes without any meaning, process-oriented coma work assumes that these signals are potentially meaningful and that we can help unfold their meaning. Any signal is a communication of some sort.

Instructions

1. **Notice and pace.** Start with noticing and pacing the comatose person's breathing and responding to any signals.

2. **Notice facial movements and expressions.** Take note of any small movements, grimaces, or expressions on the person's face.

3. **Use sculpting methods.** Use a hands-on method we call sculpting to bring awareness to processes happening in the facial muscles. In sculpting you use your hands like a sensitive sculptor or potter to sense and follow muscular feedback. This method helps the comatose person feel her facial muscles and get in contact with processes that may be happening in this area. You will also notice spontaneous facial signals from the comatose person, and help them unfold.

Here are some sculpting methods for getting in touch with experiences in the face:

❖ Gently move your fingers in a massage-like manner on the muscles of the cheeks so the person can sense any experiences happening there. Draw your fingers upward and outward, and then downward on the cheeks, noticing any responses (Figure 31).

❖ Try sculpting the person's forehead by drawing the skin to either side and then back again, noticing any responses (Figure 32).

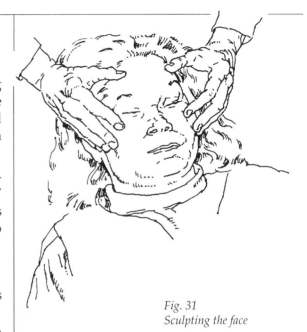
Fig. 31
Sculpting the face

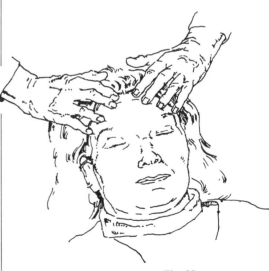
Fig. 32
Sculpting the forehead

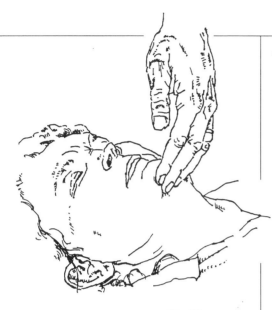

Fig. 33
Lifting the chin

❖ Put your thumb underneath the chin and lift the jaw up slightly, noticing any responses. Then press downward a bit in the opposite direction, noticing reactions and responding verbally (Figures 33 and 34).

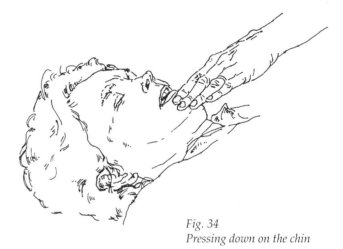

Fig. 34
Pressing down on the chin

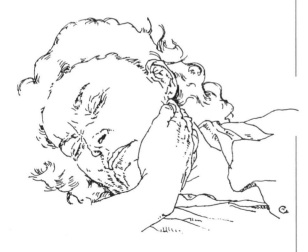

Fig. 35
Pressing forward on jawbone

Gently press forward on the jawbone, and notice any feedback (Figure 35).

Remember, you can amplify expressions by moving your hands in the direction the muscles are moving or by slightly moving them against this direction. If the person's brow is scrunched together, use your hands to mold and sculpt the forehead and eyebrows in the direction the face is moving, always noticing any responses.

If you notice spontaneous facial movements and signals, try the following:

If the cheeks, forehead, eyebrows, or chin are making slight or larger movements, follow these signals and join them with gentle sculpting motions, using your hands to accentuate facial expressions.

❖ If there are movements of the mouth, try the following.

- Rub the lips gently with your fingers.

- Put your hands on the chin, gently pressing downward and then upward, noticing any responses. The person may try to close or open her mouth.

- Gently try to open the jaw as the person inhales, then let the jaw almost shut on the exhale (Figure 36). To open the mouth, gently part the lips and place your finger and thumb between the teeth. Be careful not to get bitten. Again, this is a strong thing to do, and you should check it out with other family members before doing it.

  One person can place one hand on the upper chest (if there are no complications in the chest), pressing very slightly on the exhale and releasing on the inhale. While you do this, tell the person you know he is present.

  You can also put one hand behind the person's neck and gently squeeze in a massage-like motion as he breathes out. Try this for a few minutes.

- If the mouth is moving or making biting motions, gently experiment with opening the mouth or putting something like a swab stick between the teeth so the person can bite on it while you hold the other end (Figure 37). If sounds or motions result, join the person in these primal communications.

- If the mouth is open, you can gently press upward and then downward on the jaw and notice responses. If the mouth is closed, you can gently press downward and notice responses.

- If the mouth is open and the tongue is moving and vibrating, experiment with gently touching the tongue (make sure that your hands are clean). If you see responses such as the tongue moving, respond verbally. For example, say:

  "Wow, that tongue! Use it."

- If the person's mouth is opening and closing, use your fingers on the chin and where the jaw connects at the ear, and say:

  "Oh the mouth opens and closes, can you use your mouth to make sounds?"

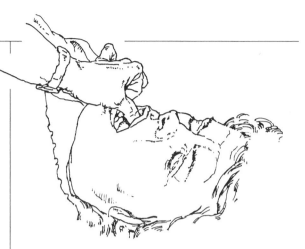

Fig. 36
Opening the mouth

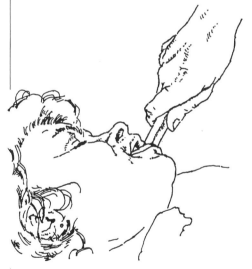

Fig. 37
Biting on a swab stick

Note: If you notice a repetitive signal, you can use this to establish binary communication (see Exercise 3 on page 97).

◦ If you notice movement of the eyelids, when the eyes are closed, rest two fingers on the eyelids and very gently move them a bit, noticing any response.

Once again, remember that in coma work, less is better. The frequency and duration of your work depend in great part on the feedback you receive from the comatose person. If your loved one seems to be responding more and more, even if subtly, and you feel you are on track, stay with what you are doing and help that experience unfold. If you receive no feedback, take a break or try another method of communication.

4. **Notice responses and encourage.** Notice any feedback to your sculpting interventions, and encourage the person to follow her experience. Use sounds and touch to deepen the experience. Say:

"Oh, yes, your forehead is moving," or

"That chin moves up and down, that means a lot to me," or

"Yes, that mouth, hmm, it's telling me something."

Working with the Face

Quick Review

1. Notice and pace the breathing.
2. Notice facial movements and expressions.
3. Use sculpting methods.
4. Notice responses and encourage the person.

Exercise 3

Asking Questions: Binary Communication

All of us have questions when someone is in a coma. Is the person in pain? Should we continue life support? What is the person experiencing? Does the person want to come out of the coma? How does she feel about her life, the possibility of her death, and the physical care she is receiving? And many more. The following method helps you ask these questions directly to the comatose person and to gain responses.

One of the most effective ways of asking questions and receiving answers from someone in a coma is to use a communication system in which the person is able to answer "yes" or "no" to questions by making a sound or a movement. We call this binary communication. You can use this form of binary communication when you are alone with the comatose person, as well as when others are around who have the same questions as you or would like to ask other questions.

Keep in mind that the person's responses may be delayed because of the amount of brain injury, the presence of drugs such as pain medication, or her momentary state. If you are unsure about the comatose person's answers to questions, try again on another day and notice any changes.

Instructions

1. **Notice and pace breathing.** Sit near the person and notice and pace the breathing. Tell the person you are there, then press the wrist on the inhalation.

2. **Notice a repetitive signal.** Setting up a binary communication system depends on identifying a repeated signal from the person. You might notice, for example, that the person repeatedly makes a tiny movement of an eyebrow, a slight movement of the mouth, a twitch of a finger, a sound, a slight turn of the head, or another signal.

3. **Establish contact using the signal.** Try to establish communication with this signal by commenting about it:

    "I notice you moving your eyebrow. You can use that eyebrow to communicate."

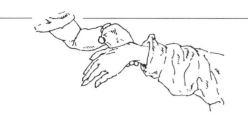

Place your hands lightly on the area where the signal originates to give the person more access to that particular signal. Wait for feedback. The next time the signal occurs, remark excitedly about it, and encourage the use of that signal to communicate.

Let's say you notice a repeated slight movement of the person's chin. You can place your hands gently on the chin to increase the person's awareness of, and access to, this signal. Or, if the person repeatedly makes a sound, you can make this sound and put your hands on the person's lips or gently on the throat. If the person slightly presses with his index finger, put your index finger next to his. Tell the person that he can use that chin motion, that sound, or that finger motion, as the case may be, to communicate if he chooses. Then wait and see whether the signal occurs again. If so, you have established communication.

Remember, if there is extensive brain injury, the person may not be able to respond easily, and responses may require time to manifest.

For a short example of this aspect of the work see the example in Chapter 9, following Exercise 5.

4. **If there is no response, try another signal or take a break.** If the person doesn't respond, wait until another signal becomes apparent. Then try again. Otherwise, relax and try another time.

5. **Set up yes-and-no communication.** Once you have established a signal of communication, set up a binary system. Tell the person that when she makes that particular signal or movement, it will mean "yes," and that no movement or response means "no." For example, imagine that the person has been raising an eyebrow. You can say:

    "You can use that signal to communicate. If you want to say yes, then move your eyebrow. If you want to say no, you needn't do anything."

    Ask if this system is okay, and watch the response. If there is a response or movement, proceed.

    If you notice that the person's head moves slightly toward you, put your cheek near her cheek and say:

    "If you want to say yes, move your head toward me just a bit. If not, you needn't move your head at all."

If the person moves her head, you have set up a binary method of communicating.

If the person gently squeezes your hand, this could be another method of communication.

Many people move their eyes. You can use the muscles around their eyes as a signal for binary communication. Touch one of the muscles at the top of the eyelids gently, and establish that the person can use her eye muscles to communicate. Say:

"You can use that muscle. Use it to say yes if you want to. Let's call a movement of that eye muscle a yes, and no movement a no. If you are in agreement, say yes now by moving this muscle again."

If she responds, you can begin to ask her questions.

6. **Ask questions about the altered state.** After you establish a signal of communication, tell the person that in a moment you will ask some questions. Give her time first to prepare inwardly. Then, speaking slowly, ask the comatose person yes-or-no questions, such as *"Are you in pain?"* Notice any responses. If the person makes the signal when you ask a particular question, then the answer is yes. If she does not respond, the answer is no. Remember that responses may be a bit delayed because of medication or physical impairment.

You will probably want to ask many questions and you should have the opportunity to do so. Many people ask questions related to ordinary concerns, such as *"Do you remember the time we went bowling together?"* or *"Is your best friend's name Tom?"* However, it is more important to ask questions related to the person's current altered state, such as:

"Are you having a good trip down there?"

"Do you want to come out?"

"Are you in pain?"

"Do you want to remain in this state?"

"Do you want to go on living?"

If you are unsure about the answers to these questions, you can wait a few days and ask the person again.

Asking Questions: Binary Communication

Quick Review

1. Notice and pace breathing.
2. Notice any repetitive signal.
3. Establish contact using the signal.
4. If there is no response, try another signal or take a break.
5. Set up yes-and-no communication.
6. Ask questions about the altered state.

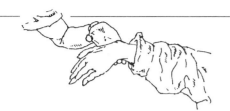

Summary of Learning from Chapter 5

❖ Notice body posture and position, and amplify through the use of your hands. Work as a team with others.

❖ Slowly move the arms, legs, shoulders, and head and notice any muscular responses.

❖ Use sculpting methods with your hands to increase the person's awareness of experiences in the musculature of the face.

❖ Develop binary communication by identifying a repetitive signal the comatose person can use to give yes-or-no answers.

Notes

1. See Arnold Mindell, *Working With the Dreaming Body,* for more on working with body signals.
2. For more information on bodywork methods see Aminah Raheem's book on process-oriented acupressure (*Process Acupressure*) and Fritz Smith's *Inner Bridges: Zero Balancing.*

Chapter 6

T he following exercises help you develop additional skills for working with people who are in comas attributable to structural brain injury and enhance and deepen the work you have been doing until this point.

In an ordinary state of consciousness, a person is able to move his body in a more or less coordinated fashion. For example, a person can use both hands simultaneously. If the person wants to turn his head to the side, he is generally able to turn other parts of the body to the side as well. However, this flawless partnership of the hands or the whole body may be disrupted by injury to the brain.

People who have suffered brain injury may be frustrated by not being able to express themselves as fully as they once did. If the person is coming closer and closer to everyday consciousness, it can be an especially frustrating experience to be unable to use parts of the body in coordination with one another. Some people with brain injury may have their full mental abilities intact, yet won't be able to get their foot or hand or another body part to follow in chorus.

The methods described in this chapter help the person get in touch with movements she may be able to imagine but not yet have the motor or vocal apparatus to execute outwardly. This work also facilitates reconnection between distant body parts, such as the head and the foot, one hand with the other, or the arms with the head.

Always try to follow the person's natural process. Notice what the comatose person is already doing, or notice responses that you receive through touching and moving the person, as described in the earlier chapters, and assist him in expressing himself congruently—that is, using his whole body in a unified way.

Exercise 2 specifically addresses working with others as a team. This type of coma work requires the ability to reach distant body parts that one person cannot manage alone. Doing coma work with others provides much-needed support and assistance. Teamwork also gives family and friends the feeling that you are doing something meaningful together and connecting in a deep way to your loved one. See the short case example in Chapter 12, Exercise 5, for an example of this. (For additional methods for working with brain-injured individuals, which are best performed with the assistance of a coma helper or therapist, see Chapter 13, Exercises 2 and 3.)

Remember, again, that doing less is best. Try one method and notice the feedback. If you get more response and good feedback, continue with what you are doing. If you do not receive much feedback, try another method or take a break. Do not overload the person with too much input.

In Exercise 3 you focus on the experience of paralysis. When someone is paralyzed on one side, there are two processes happening simultaneously. One is paralysis, the other is mobility. You will focus first on one of these experiences and then on the other.

While all of us want the quickest results, bear in mind that it is quite normal for work with brain-injured individuals to take more time and require more patience than work with individuals in comas with metabolic origins. If possible, find others who can encourage, love, and support you, and invite family and friends to assist you.

Exercise 1

Reconnecting Parts

In this exercise you try to connect movements of parts of the face, head, and neck with the breath and sounds. These methods you can perform alone. Exercise 2 requires the assistance of others to make connections throughout the body.

Instructions

1. **Approach the person.** Once again, approach the person by pacing her breathing, speaking on the exhale. Touch the person's wrist in conjunction with the breath. Encourage the person to follow and believe in her experiences. Mention sensory-oriented channels, and notice responses.

2. **Respond to minimal signals.** Test body parts, notice responses, and respond with sounds and blank-access statements. Notice the mood the person is in (for example, relaxed or wakeful). Make sure your responses mirror these signals in quality and tempo.

3. **Notice any movements of the mouth, jaw, head, neck, or breath.** Notice any motions, even if minimal, of the mouth, the jaw, the head, or the neck, or notice whether the breath is the most outstanding signal. Respond with sound or touch.

4. **Discover connections.** Amplify these experiences. Make connections that help the person recall coordinated movement or the ability to make sounds, or both. Following are some helpful tips.

❖ If the neck and head tend to turn to the side:
  ▫ Place one of your hands on the jawbone and the other hand on the back of the neck. Gently experiment with moving the head and jaw in the same direction and in the same rhythm as the original movement. This is effective because muscles in the back of the neck are closely connected to the jaw (Figure 38).

❖ If breathing is the main signal:
  ▫ Gently rest your hands on the person's chest or stomach. Slightly press on the exhale, and release the pressure on the inhale. Hum a simple children's song that goes along with this rhythm.

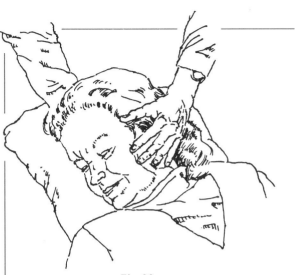

Fig. 38
Moving the head and jaw

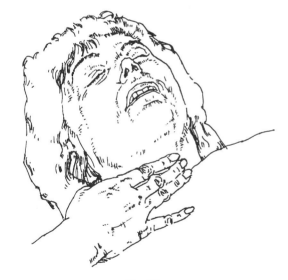

Fig. 39
Fingers on the Adam's apple in association with sound

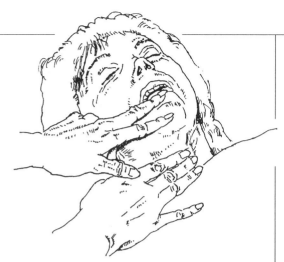

Fig. 40
Fingers on the Adam's apple and mouth in association with sound

- Gently squeeze the back of the head or neck in rhythm with the exhalation. Make sounds that go along with this rhythm.

❖ If the mouth quivers or moves:

  - A basic connection that we have all developed is the relationship between the hands and the mouth. If the mouth is moving, you can lightly touch the lips and simultaneously gently squeeze one of the hands in rhythm with these mouth movements.

  - Mouth movements may be connected with the desire to make sounds. Here are some methods for connecting sound and mouth motions.

    - Put one or two of your fingers gently on the person's lips. Say that you notice her lip movements and that you are listening. Then place your fingers lightly on the person's Adam's apple (Figure 39). Make a sound, and tell the comatose person that this is the location from which sound comes. Tell her that she can also make noises in conjunction with her mouth motions while gently touching the lips and Adam's apple simultaneously (Figure 40).

    - Place your fingers on the chin and where the jaw connects at the ear, and say:

      "Oh, the mouth opens and closes. Can you use your mouth to make sounds?"

    - If the mouth moves with or without sounds, place one of the comatose person's hands on her own chest. Then put one of your hands on top of hers. Tell her that these areas are connected, that sounds and chest motions go together, and that she can use them both to make sounds.

    - Still another way of reinforcing the person's contact with her own sounds is to place your lips on the person's head and make vibratory sounds while blowing gently.

❖ Notice the pulse. Notice whether its rate is fast or slow. Tap very lightly on the head and the back of the neck in the rhythm of the pulse.

5. **Notice feedback.** Notice when you get the most feedback, and amplify the process as it unfolds.

Reconnecting Parts

Quick Review

1. **Approach the person.**
2. **Respond to minimal signals.**
3. **Identify the strongest signal.**
4. **Discover connections.**
5. **Notice any feedback.**

Exercise 2

Working with Others

In this exercise you work together with others to facilitate connection among the comatose person's body parts. Working as a team makes it possible to apply many methods you are unable to perform alone. For example, with the help of other family members and friends, you can connect simultaneously with various parts of the person's body that one person cannot reach alone. Also, another team worker's eyes can help you notice signals that you may miss when you are focusing on one part of the person's body.

In this exercise you will find many different possible modes of interacting. Be sure to try one method at a time, and notice the feedback. If you get responses to what you are doing, remain with that particular method of communicating for a short time, then pause. If you do not get much response, try a different method or take a break. Do not overload the person by trying too many methods in succession.

First, read through the instructions alone. Then explain them to others, or read them together as a team. Use the steps summarized in the box following this exercise as a guide when you work with the comatose person.

Instructions

1. **Approach the person.** As always, one person should begin by pacing the breath and encouraging the person to believe in his experiences. Mention the sensory channels, and notice any responses.

2. **Mention that others are present.** Your team workers can join the person's breathing by gently touching and pressing on the wrist, head, and balls of the feet, one at a time, and watching for feedback.

3. **Respond to minimal signals.** Use sounds and blank-access statements in response to any signals. Then, someone can test body parts and notice responses.

4. **Identify the strongest signal.** What is the strongest signal you notice? Where is it happening? Is it the breath? A sound? A movement?

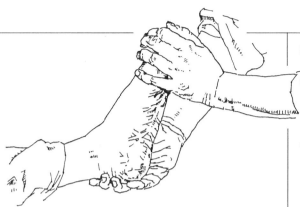

Fig. 41
*Gently pressing and
extending balls and heel of
foot to rhythm of breath*

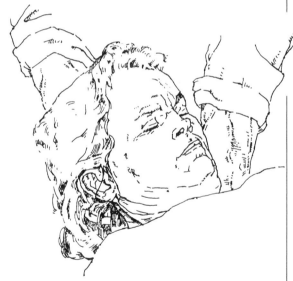

Fig. 42
*Lifting head up and
down to breathing rate*

5. **Discover connections.** Now try to connect this signal to other body parts. Use the others in your group to help establish a sense of congruency throughout the comatose person's body. Following are tips you can use with particular body signals. Remember to use sounds that mirror the quality of the person's signals.

❖ Notice and work with the breath.
  ▫ Breathe rhythmically with the person as you rest your hands on the person's chest or stomach, slightly pressing on the exhale and lifting on the inhale.

  One family member can press gently on the back of the person's head or neck in rhythm with the exhalation.

  Another person can press slightly on the balls of the feet as the person inhales, and pull gently backward on the back of the heels as the person exhales (Figure 41).

  Everyone can hum or speak in this rhythm.

  ▫ Another variation: Gently lift the head up (inhalation) and down (exhalation), mirroring the rate of breathing. Support the upper back and base of the head with one hand, using the other hand as a cradle for the head (Figure 42).

  Meanwhile, another person can gently lift the eyelids (just a fractional amount) to this rhythm. At another point, others can lift the arms and legs to this rhythm; lift all the limbs at once in conjunction with breathing, and make sounds or hum to this rhythm.

❖ If the person squeezes your hand:
  ▫ Squeeze the person's hand back. Others can gently squeeze her shoulders, the leg, or the other hand.
❖ If the hand slightly jitters:
  ▫ Gently wobble the other hand, the knees, or the feet.

- ❖ If one arm is moving about, and if the movement is slow:
    - ▫ Move the head gently in conjunction with this spontaneous arm motion (Figure 43).
    - ▫ Move the second arm in conjunction with the first arm (Figure 44).
    - ▫ Then add the legs, moving them as above (Figure 45).

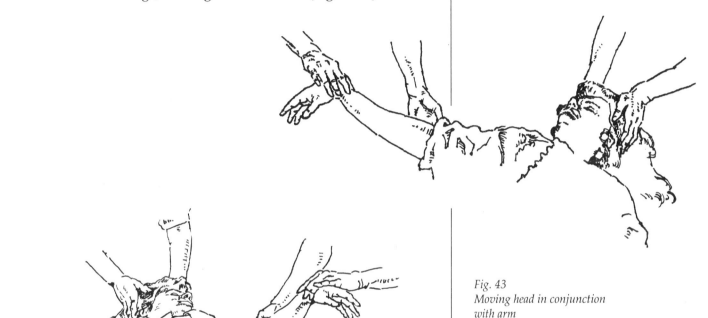

Fig. 43
Moving head in conjunction with arm

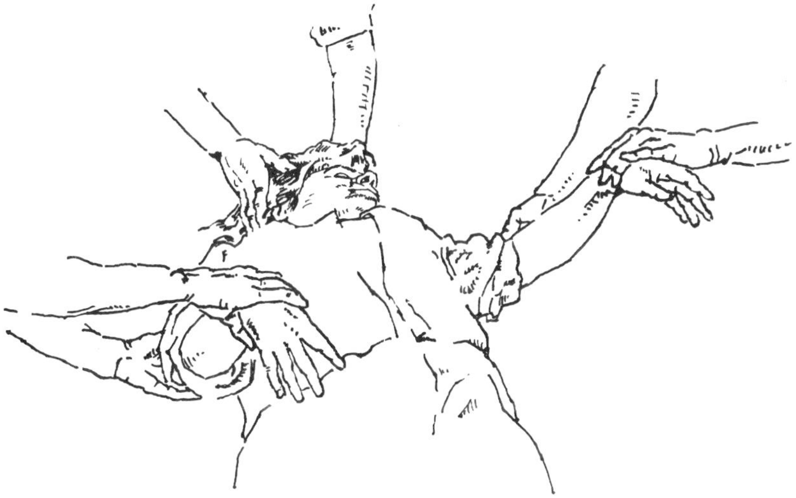

Fig. 44
Moving other arm as well

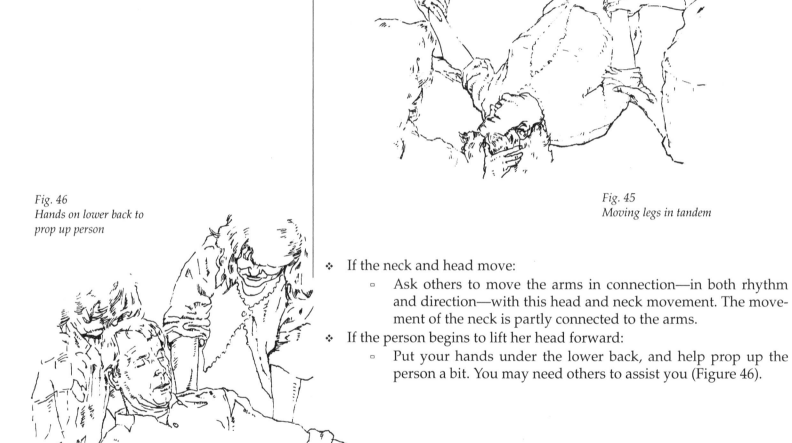

Fig. 46
Hands on lower back to prop up person

Fig. 45
Moving legs in tandem

❖ If the neck and head move:
   ▫ Ask others to move the arms in connection—in both rhythm and direction—with this head and neck movement. The movement of the neck is partly connected to the arms.
❖ If the person begins to lift her head forward:
   ▫ Put your hands under the lower back, and help prop up the person a bit. You may need others to assist you (Figure 46).

❖ If one foot or the head (or both) falls to one side:

   ▫ With the help of others, gently move the whole body in this direction to the side. Do the same thing if the knee is also bent and extended to the side (Figure 47). If the person curls up in a fetal position, join with others to stroke the back and head, comforting her. Sing a soothing song.

6. **Notice any feedback.** Notice where and when you get the most feedback, and amplify the process as it deepens and unfolds.

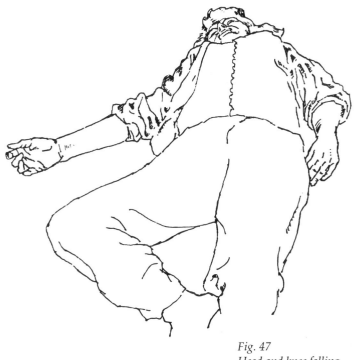

Fig. 47
*Head and knee falling
to the side*

Working with Others

Quick Review
1. **Approach the person.**
2. **Mention that others are present.**
3. **Respond to minimal signals.**
4. **Identify the strongest signal.**
5. **Discover connections.**
6. **Notice any feedback.**

Exercise 3

One Side Teaches the Other

If one side or part of the person's body is paralyzed as a result of brain injury, special methods enable the comatose person to experience a sense of unity throughout the body and aid with the recuperation process.

The core approach in these methods is to acknowledge that there are *two* processes happening simultaneously in the person. One process involves the lack of ordinary activity, or paralysis. We say that this body part is "dreaming," and coma methods involve following and unfolding the experiences of this part of the body. It may seem strange to encourage the "dreaming" aspect of these body parts, instead of trying to get them to recuperate. Yet, we have found that if the experiences of the impaired side of the body are followed and validated, this, paradoxically, has a recuperative effect on the body as a whole. When validated, these experiences do not have to disrupt the body but instead tend to generate overall recuperation.

The second method focuses on using the recuperative powers of the unimpaired side of the body. This side of the body is used as a teacher of healing and recuperation for the paralyzed side. Here, the "healthy" side of the body teaches the paralyzed side how to function once again. This method is a well-known procedure in the medical field.[1]

Which process you follow depends on feedback. Try one method. If you receive strong feedback, stay with it. If not, try the other method. This may change within one session or over time. As with all of these methods, time and patience are necessary.

This exercise explores both methods. For ease in the description of the exercise, I am calling one side of the body "unimpaired" and the other side "paralyzed".

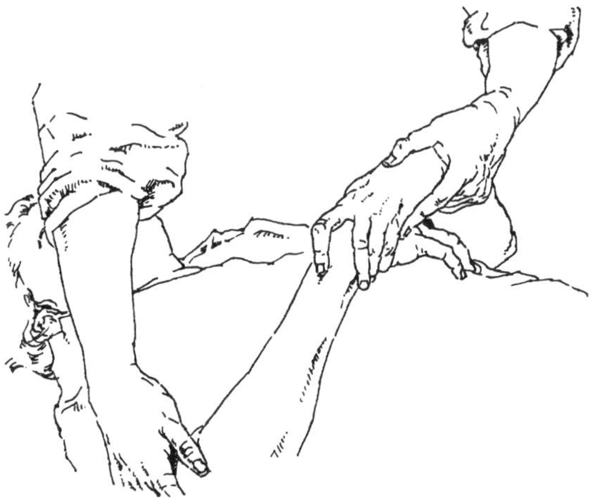

Instructions

1. **Help the unimpaired hand teach the paralyzed hand.** Begin with the unimpaired hand. When you see it move, take it and gently help it to grasp the hand that is paralyzed (Figure 48). Say simply:

   "Your right hand is holding your left" (or vice versa).

Fig. 48
"Unimpaired" hand moves the "paralyzed" hand

Move the impaired hand around with this hand. You are using the "awake" hand to interact with the "sleepy" hand.

Then guide both hands to the face. Use the unimpaired hand to help the paralyzed hand feel the person's own face, cheeks, and lips (Figure 49). As you do this, say something like:

"This is your face, your lips, and your right [or left] hand is teaching you this."

2. **Now start with the paralyzed hand.** Pick up the hand that is impaired and say:

"This is your left [or right] hand."

Then help it pick up the "unimpaired" hand, saying:

"This is your other hand. You are holding both together."

You can also pick up the paralyzed hand yourself and bring it up to the person's face. Say what you are doing as you help the impaired hand to feel the person's own face. For example, put the hand on the person's lips, rubbing them gently, and say:

"These are your lips, your eyebrows," and so forth…

3. **Notice any feedback.** Notice any feedback you get from the comatose person, and mirror it with sound and touch.

4. **Support the process of the impaired arm or hand.** Discover the process in the impaired arm by gently lifting it and moving it slightly, as described in Chapter 5, Exercise 1. When you discover the experience in this arm, help the person experience this in other parts of his body. Here are suggestions:

❖ If the limb is flaccid and relaxed, encourage the comatose person to amplify the relaxation of paralysis. You might say:

"Just relax, yes… vacation… you don't have to do anything at all."

Use gentle touch on various parts of the body to help the person sense this relaxation in the whole body, including the other arm.

❖ If the paralyzed side of the body is not simply relaxed, but expresses another type of process, see if you can help the unimpaired arm express this process, as explained in Chapter 5, Exercise 1.

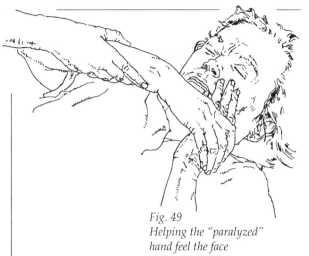

Fig. 49
Helping the "paralyzed" hand feel the face

One Side Teaches the Other

Quick Review

1. Help the unimpaired hand teach the other hand.
2. Now start with the impaired hand.
3. Notice any feedback.
4. Support the process of the impaired arm.

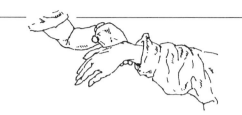

Summary of Learning from Chapter 6

❖ Assist the comatose person's natural process by noticing signals he is already making. Help him experience and express himself congruently through the body by connecting body parts. You can do this alone or with the help of others.

❖ Notice and help create connections between the neck, the head, the arms and legs, and the breath.

❖ Remember that when someone is paralyzed on one side, there are two processes happening simultaneously: one is paralysis, the other is more or less normal. Support both of these experiences.

❖ Work with the paralysis experience by encouraging the person to relax, to not do anything, or to follow the "dreaming" experiences in that part of the body.

❖ Help the unimpaired hand of the body teach the paralyzed side. Use the unimpaired hand to help the paralyzed hand feel and become re-acquainted with the person's own face, cheeks, and lips.

❖ Remember that doing less is best. Follow the feedback. If the person seems to respond to what you are doing, continue; if not, try a different method or take a break.

Note

1. See Bobath, *Abnormal Postural Reflex Activity Caused by Brain Lesions.* The observation that two processes are happening in the body simultaneously, and supporting each of these, are new contributions from process work.

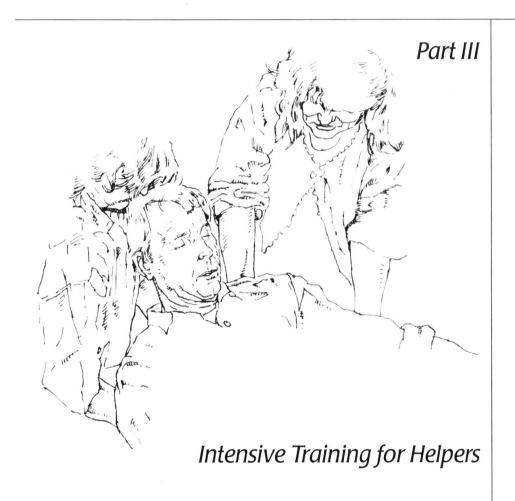

Part III

Intensive Training for Helpers

hapters 7 through 14 provide practical training exercises and self-explorative work for:

- Helping professionals and students needing an intensive training program they can follow in a classroom or in small learning groups.

- Family members and friends of comatose individuals who would like to practice and learn more extensive coma work and try personal exercises.

Exercise Sequence

Some of the exercises in this section focus on the helper's personal development; others move toward developing specific skills and feeling qualities for working with people in any kind of coma. Chapters 12 and 13 address skills specifically aimed at working with people in comas resulting from brain injury. Many of those exercises call for the participation of three or more people. Take time to learn all the methods. The fundamental principles introduced in Chapter 12 for use with people in structural comas are generally helpful for all types of coma. The summary exercises in Chapter 14 will help you assimilate what you are learning.

For learning purposes, I have developed individual coma work exercises. However, once you are familiar with these methods, they will no longer seem so separate. Instead, they will form a collection of tools allowing you to respond to the momentary situation and follow the individual's process. You will begin to communicate in a more fluid way as you feel more comfortable with, and adept at, following the comatose person's experiences and signals. As you interact with the comatose person, you will gain a sense of the direction the process is taking, and this sense of direction, rather than following a set of techniques, will become your guide.

Remember, when you are with someone in a coma, the first step is to make certain that all medical problems have been taken care of as much as possible. Then, begin your work.

If you are a relative or friend of someone in a coma and you have been practicing the fundamental coma exercises in Part II with the comatose person, you can supplement your learning by trying the following exercises with other family members and friends when you feel you have the time. Following these exercises may help you with your personal feelings and emotional states, give you additional practice, and help you gain a more profound understanding of what it may be like to be in a coma. You will then be able to apply these skills to your communication with the comatose person. You will also be able to work on your own inner processes and development.

For classroom situations, I suggest meeting one or two times a week for two-and-a-half or three-hour periods. During each class, try two or three exercises, depending on time, energy, and the participants' ability to absorb new information. Although the exercises proceed in a linear fashion, I recommend that you alternate the exercises that concern the helpers' personal work (Chapters 7 and 10) with more skill-oriented exercises (Chapters 8, 9, 11, 12, and 13). Finish your studies with the integration exercises in Chapter 14. Take time between exercises to discuss theory and readings, answer questions, and talk about personal experiences and learning.

I have included time allocations for each exercise to create a framework for these experiences. However, the length of each exercise can be altered depending on the experiences and needs of the group. It is helpful to mention to the person in the "comatose" state, at the appropriate time, that there are only a few minutes remaining in the exercise. That way, she will begin to prepare inwardly for the emergence from the altered state. She will have time to adjust to ordinary reality and to talk about her personal experiences and will be able to give you, the helper, feedback about your work.

If possible, videotape one or more of the exercises in which one person imagines that she is in a deep trance or comatose state while her partner tries various coma work methods. In the next class meeting the videotape can be very helpful as a learning tool for noticing various elements of coma work. See Chapter 11, Exercise 4, for guidelines on watching the videotape.

Class Responses and Examples

After a few of the exercises, I have provided responses from my class participants about their own experiences with these exercises. In addition, when possible, I have included examples either from actual work with a comatose person or from demonstrations in training seminars illustrating skills to be learned in a particular exercise.

Doing the Exercises

Most of the exercises in this section require the participation of two people. One person acts as the helper while the other person is either interviewed about issues related to coma work or imagines that she is in a deep trance or comatose state. After half of the allotted time, switch roles so that each person has a full experience of being the helper and the "comatose" person.

The person imagining that she is in a comatose state should lie down on the floor, couch, bed, or massage table. If she is on the floor, it is a bit more difficult physically for the coma helper, but he can sit right next to her and work from this position as well. Most of my classes have been conducted in this fashion on the floor.

If at any time during the exercise you, as the "comatose" person, feel afraid or do not want to continue, tell the helper to stop and take some time to discuss what has happened. If you (or any participant) are shy about lying down, you can also lean back in a chair. If you do not want to do a particular exercise, watch others as they practice. You can gain a lot through observation. The personal work exercises may also help you with your fears and inner processes.

Discussing Your Work

At the end of each exercise, I suggest that you discuss the exercise with your practice partner. The best form of learning, I have found, is direct, compassionate feedback from the person who is acting as if she were in a comatose state. What was helpful and what would have been more helpful? Take time to discuss learning and discoveries.

After each exercise, also discuss the "comatose" person's inner experiences. Since we are dealing with deep altered states, significant personal experiences may arise during the exercises, experiences that may be quite new for you. You may discover feelings and images that are surprising to you. Or you might find yourself inside experiences that feel "unusually" familiar, yet have been far away from your ordinary consciousness. The best way to integrate and ground the experiences before getting up is to take time to discuss the possible meaning of these experiences for your everyday life.

Personal Log

I provide blank pages at the back of this book to record your experiences and learning. Use these pages or begin a journal of your own. Save these notes. You can look back at them at any time to recall what you have discovered personally and practically.

Additional Learning

It is helpful to learn as much as you can about anatomy, physiology, and medical procedures, although I do not discuss these topics in this book. Find books and study materials, and look at pictures of muscular and skeletal systems (see the Bibliography for references).

The Metaskill of Learning

As you practice the various skills and metaskills (feeling qualities), they will become more familiar and easier to apply. Your work will develop increasing fluidity, always welcome after the inevitably awkward beginning stages. Some of you will feel that you have been doing this work your whole lifetime. Others may need time to find your own comfort and expression through the coma work. Remember that all of us are learning how to communicate with people in coma. Be patient with yourself. In time, this way of interacting will become second nature. Treat yourself with as much love and patience as you would offer anyone else.

Relaxing

Sometimes coma work can be tiring, especially if you are standing for a long time. Make yourself as comfortable as possible. When you are with a comatose person, stand next to the bed, sit on a chair, or sit on the side of the bed if that is appropriate. Don't wear yourself out. Wear comfortable clothes and shoes if possible. Take a break, have tea. Do not remain in one body position for too long. Change position, adjust your back, or take a walk. Discuss what has been happening with others who are there. Talk to the family.

Teaching Family and Friends

After you have learned these methods, it is helpful to share them with family and friends of the comatose person. In this way, those close to the comatose person can use these methods to communicate with their loved one and continue the work when you are not present.

Remember to talk with the parents and family. Give them time to talk about themselves, their fears, the shock, their worries. One parent said that just having someone listen to him with a compassionate ear was a huge relief.

Coma Work Tips

When you work with a comatose person, there are a number of things to remember, including the following:

❖ **Talk to staff, and keep relatives informed.** In her article on coma work and nursing, Kay Ross suggests that you talk to the nursing staff, invite their questions, and find out when is the best time to visit. Ask about medical equipment if you do not understand it. Keep relatives informed about your coma work.[1]

❖ **Know that less is best.** Remember that in coma work, less is best. Follow the feedback. If the person seems to respond to what you are doing, continue on that path. If you do not get a response, try another method or take a break. If you find yourself getting sleepy, this may be an indication that either you or the comatose person, or both of you, needs a rest.

❖ **The type of responses and interactions that you make should mirror the quality and rhythm of the signals of the comatose person.** The way that you interact depends on the responses and feedback of the comatose person. Sometimes your work unfolds into broad movements and sounds, and at other times it is minute and subtle.

Know that even the most slight, subtle interactions on your part which are done with care and are related to the comatose person's quiet inner state can connect deeply with him. On the other hand, while it is natural to always be quiet when we are with someone in such a deep altered state of consciousness, you can afford to be more expressive if the quality of the person's signals is more intense and energetic. In that way the comatose person will feel more related to.

❖ **Recognize your own trancelike feelings.** During the course of your work as the helper, you may find yourself falling into a light trance or dreamy state. This is quite natural, since you are attempting to align yourself with the comatose person's state of consciousness. During this state, fantasies may arise.

While in general it is most beneficial to simply follow the signals of the comatose person without interpreting them, in this case you might experiment, mentioning your fantasies to the comatose person. Make sure, however, to notice the feedback. If you seem to get responses to these fantasies, continue on this track. Elaborate verbally on particular words or images that the person responds to. If you do not receive a response, try another method or take a break. (See Chapter 11, Exercise 7, for more on using your intuition.)

❖ **Keep a log of signals and experiences.** When you do work with a comatose person, keep a log of signals and events that may be linked with feedback from the comatose person. For example, you may notice that the person responds strongly when a certain person comes into the room, or when his dog is brought in! Perhaps he gives a strong response when special music that he loves is played or when you touch his finger or pace his breathing. Note the signals and events and the types of responses. You may be able to use these responses as a means of communication, to elicit answers to questions from the comatose person. (See Chapter 9, Exercise 5, on binary communication.)

Note

1. Ross, "A Comparison of the Medical/Nursing and Process Work Approaches to Coma."

Chapter 7

C oma training cannot be separated from learning about your own altered states and your feelings about life and death. The following exercises will help prepare you inwardly for coma work and will help you understand more deeply the inner processes of comatose individuals. The more empathy and understanding you have with the comatose person, the better your work will be.

Also, for you personally, practicing these methods is a form of preventive medicine. The more varied and rich your experiences are, the less likely it is that injury or ill health will surprise you by occurring unexpectedly.

Note: Each exercise includes a detailed description followed by a short summation of steps. Become acquainted with the description first, and then use the summary to guide you as you work.

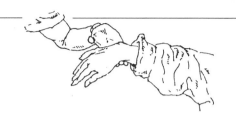

EXERCISES

Exercise 1

Why Do You Want to Do this Work?

At the beginning of each of my courses, I ask participants why they want to train in coma work. Your answer to this question is relevant to your own development and informs the way you accompany comatose people. You may want to refer to this answer again when you have progressed further in the book.

Instructions *(in pairs; 10 minutes per person; interview one another)*

1. **Discuss why you want to study coma work.** What motivates you? Identify personal, professional, and spiritual reasons.

2. **Write down your answers.** Use the pages in the back of this book to write down your responses. You will return to this question at the end of your studies, to review and update your answer.

Common responses to the question in this exercise, collected from my class participants, include the following:

❖ To communicate with family members or friends in comatose states.

❖ To improve skills as a nurse, doctor, hospice volunteer, or caretaker.

❖ To reach the deepest part of people.

❖ To learn to communicate with people in altered states of consciousness.

❖ To find out more about my own altered states of consciousness.

❖ To help increase my skills in working with people in normal states of consciousness.

❖ To learn to trust my perceptions and inner feelings.

❖ To be of service to people who do not have a "voice."

❖ To know more about the breadth and depth of human experience.

Why Do You Want to Do this Work?
Quick Review
1. **Discuss why you want to study coma work.**
2. **Write down your answers.**

Exercise 2

Lying Down

Coma is the result of mechanical difficulties; it is also a call for inner work. We have learned that people in comatose states are in need of time to process internal experiences without the distractions of every-day life.

One of the best ways to take a glimpse of the world of coma is to experiment with your own internal states. In this way you not only have a chance to feel more deeply what this experience could be like for someone in a coma, but also may find out more about yourself.

The following exercise can be done alone, with a partner guiding you, or with one member of the class leading everyone through the exercise simultaneously.

Instructions (*in pairs; 5 to 10 minutes per person*)

1. **Lie down on the floor.** Relax and imagine yourself in a coma or a deep trance state.

2. **Take a couple of minutes.** Allow yourself to sink into and simply be in that state for a couple of minutes.

3. **Ask yourself a question.** Now ask yourself the following question: Is there anything useful about this state? Does it evoke any quality or feeling that you need or normally don't have?

4. **Explore your feelings.** Spend a few minutes exploring this question as you remain lying on the floor. When you are ready, relate your feelings to a partner.

5. **Write down your answers.** Take time to write down your answers to the questions.

Responses to the question "Does this state evoke any quality or feeling you need?" gathered from class participants include the following:

❖ Healing.
❖ Relief from exhaustion.
❖ A deep sense of myself.

Lying Down

Quick Review
1. **Lie down on the floor.**
2. **Take a few minutes.**
3. **Ask yourself a question.**
4. **Explore your feelings.**
5. **Write down your answers.**

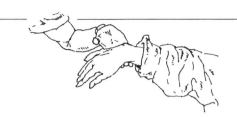

- ❖ A sense of detachment.
- ❖ A time to take a break from doing lots of things.
- ❖ A sense of letting go of responsibility.
- ❖ Getting in touch with myself and my feelings.
- ❖ Deep peace.
- ❖ Connection with love.
- ❖ A letting go of inhibitions.
- ❖ A sense of getting away from ordinary life, people, home, work, and so forth.

Coma Work and Edges

All over the world, we have found central growing edges that emerge in students learning coma work. Edges are blocks or barriers. You are at an edge when you feel that you cannot go further, or that you are shy, afraid, or inhibited about the next step. The edge stands between your known identity and unknown experiences. Over the edge we discover new aspects of ourselves.

Central edges of the coma work student include the following:

- ❖ Shyness about and awkwardness in assisting someone who is in an altered state of consciousness.
- ❖ Fear about one's own altered states.
- ❖ Fear of death.
- ❖ Inhibitions about being expressive with sound, touch, and movement.
- ❖ Fear and shyness about intimacy and contact.

For some of you, coma work feels natural. You feel at home with this kind of intimate and loving communication—perhaps even more than you do relating in more ordinary ways. However, for those of us who still have edges, blocks, or shyness, let's start with an exercise on our own altered states. (Exercises on other personal edges can be found in Chapter 8.

Exercise 3

Working on Your Own Altered States

Sometimes we are uncomfortable working with people in comatose states because we feel out of touch with, or embarrassed about, our own altered states of consciousness. Many of the altered states we all go through at one time or another are so foreign to our ordinary identities that we try to cut them off or hide them. Some of us are driven to search for them in addictive substances, relationships, or other means. More awareness of our own altered states gives us deep knowledge of ourselves. It also gives us a better understanding of what people may be experiencing in deep trance states and creates a greater sense of ease in working with comatose people.

Without knowledge of our own altered states, it is difficult to grasp and follow the experiences that someone may be having in a coma. This exercise helps us bridge a gap between ourselves and individuals in coma by giving us the feeling that we have, in some way, "been there, too"—that deep trance and comatose states are really not that foreign to us. Try the following interview and exercise with a partner.

Instructions *(in pairs; 20 minutes per person; one person interviews and works with the other, then reverse)*

Interview

1. **Remember an altered state.** Recall one time in your life when you were in a strongly altered state of consciousness (possibly as a result of illness, drugs, relationship difficulties in which an altered state emerged from being passionately in love or full of anger, an accident, a coma, ecstasy, or another experience). What was it like? Describe this state to your partner.

2. **Describe relationships.** What were your relationships like with other people during this time? Did you feel:

❖ That you didn't need other people?
❖ That others were helpful?
❖ That others could not communicate with you or did not understand you?

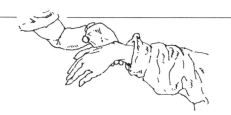

Exercise

3. **Explore the altered state.** If you were to explore or in some way complete this altered state, what would be most helpful to you? With the help of your partner, experiment with expressing that state in movement or sound, or in visual fantasy. Stay with this experience until you discover whether there is a message the altered state is trying to express.

If you are afraid of the altered state, ask your partner to act it out for you as you look on. Tell her which movements and sounds to make that express your altered state. For example, one woman's altered state was a moment of ecstasy. She described this ecstatic feeling as the sun shining brightly and warmly down upon her and the Earth. She asked her partner to act like the sun by raising her arms up to the sky and then opening them slowly and widely to the side.

Continue to choreograph the movements and sounds that your partner makes until you find out whether there is a message that the altered state is expressing.

4. **Discuss with your partner.** Can you bring the message from your altered state into everyday reality somehow? If not, why not?

5. **Write down your experiences.** Take time to write your experiences in your personal log at the end of the book.

Working on Your Own Altered States

Quick Review

    Interview

1. Remember an altered state.
2. Describe relationships.

    Exercise

3. Explore the altered state.
4. Discuss with your partner.
5. Write down your experiences.

Exercise 4

The Meaning of Life

For many of us, working with people in comatose states reminds us of our longing to discover and stay close to the very essence and meaning of our own lives. What is my life really about? What is most important to me? The following exercise helps you get in contact with essential elements of your own life and, it is hoped, helps you lessen the gap between yourself and the comatose person.

Instructions *(alone or guided by a class member; 10 minutes)*

1. **Sit quietly in a comfortable position.** Sit on a chair or on the floor and get comfortable. Take some time to be quietly with yourself.

2. **Imagine that you have six months to live.** Consider the possibility that you just heard you have only six months more to live.

3. **Consider what is important to you.** If you knew you were going to die in six months, what would you feel? What would be most important to you? What things might you give up? What would you do? Consider work, creativity, inner life, relationships, and so forth.

4. **Note feelings in your head.** Notice whether answering the above questions has any effect on the feelings in your head. Does your head feel different than before? In this exercise some people sense that the head is broadening, dissolving, warming, opening up, giving up effort, or getting lighter.

5. **Write notes.** Write down answers to the questions in No. 3 above.

The Meaning of Life

Quick Review

1. Sit quietly in a comfortable position.
2. Imagine that you have six months live.
3. Consider what is important to you.
4. Note feelings in your head.
5. Write notes.

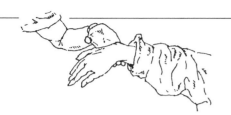

Exercise 5

Exploring Your Feelings about Death

For many of us, coma work brings up our own feelings, views, and concerns about death. Your conscious or unconscious beliefs about death affect your interactions with someone who is in a coma or in a near-death condition, or both, whether or not you are aware of these beliefs. Identifying your own beliefs is important for understanding the reactions you may have when you are working with a comatose person.

Awareness of your beliefs is also helpful because, once you know them, you can stand back and notice what is actually happening with the comatose person. Try the following exercise.

Instructions (*in pairs; 10 minutes per person*)

1. **Talk about your feelings.** How do you feel about death? Do you feel scared? Is it exciting, agonizing, or painful?

2. **Discuss experiences.** What experiences have you had with family members or friends who have died?

3. **Mention personal experiences.** Have you personally had experiences with death? Mention any near-death experiences, serious accidents, illnesses, or the like.

4. **Share your feelings about what happens after death.** What are your beliefs about what happens after death? Do you have personal, spiritual, or religious beliefs? Do you believe in an afterlife?

5. **Discuss answers.** Talk about your answers and feelings with your partner.

Exploring Your Feelings about Death

Quick Review

1. Talk about your feelings.
2. Discuss experiences.
3. Mention your personal experiences.
4. Share your feelings about what happens after death.
5. Discuss answers.

Exercise 6

Imagining Death and New Life

Many people are afraid of death. This fear often appears during stressful times such as midlife crises or at other critical periods in our lives because, symbolically, some part of us wants to die in order for other aspects of ourselves to be born. At such times, aspects of one's self-identity feel worn out. Don Juan, the Yaqui Indian shaman in Carlos Castenada's books, speaks of death as an ally that brings us close to our very essence. He says that knowing your death is the way to become "real" as opposed to being a "phantom," that is, merely a person who has adapted solely to consensus reality.

Try this exercise in which you fantasize that "you" die, noticing which part of you would like to drop away and which parts would like to be born.

Instructions (*in pairs, guided by your partner; 10 minutes per person*)

1. **Recall fear of death.** Remember one time in your life when you were afraid of death.

2. **Imagine part of yourself dying.** Lie down. Let go and relax, and imagine which part of you needs to "die."

3. **Find out which part wants to live.** Ask yourself which part is still here. Which part wants to live?

4. **Be this part.** Still lying down, let yourself be this new part. Feel it in your body. Imagine living this way in the world.

5. **Notice any impulse to move.** Now wait until you notice any movement that starts to happen in your body.

6. **Follow the impulse into life.** Follow this movement as it brings you back into life.

7. **Discover more about this part.** Discover how this new part of you would like to live. What would change? How would you be different?

8. **Discuss and take notes.** Talk about your experience with your partner, and write notes about your experiences.

Imagining Death and New Life

Quick Review

1. Recall fear of death.
2. Imagine part of yourself dying.
3. Find out which part wants to live.
4. Be this part.
5. Notice any impulse to move.
6. Follow impulse into life.
7. Discover more about this part.
8. Discuss and take notes.

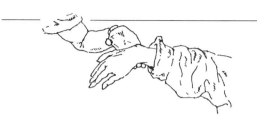

Exercise 7

Inner Work Basics

Coma work is based on your ability to follow and assist someone in her deep inner state. To heighten your sensitivity and abilities to do this, it is most helpful to learn to follow and appreciate your own internal experiences.

In this exercise you learn a basic method for working on yourself. You learn about your internal processes and gain a greater appreciation of the comatose person's inner experiences and methods for helping those experiences unfold.

Knowing how to follow your own internal states can be very important for you. Much of the fear of dying is related to the dread of being trapped in inner vegetative states that we are unable to make use of or follow. Experience has shown that people who value and learn how to follow their inner experiences are able to use their awareness in a more useful way if they do fall into a vegetative state. Therefore, not only for your work with others but to alleviate your own fears of these states, try the following training method. You can use this exercise at any time to get in contact with your inner experiences and replenish yourself!

Sensory-Oriented Experience

Process-oriented inner work[1] helps us become aware of the flow of our inner experience by noticing the sensory-oriented channel in which our process is occurring. *Sensory-oriented* means that these experiences are occurring through the various sensory modalities, such as hearing, feeling, seeing, or moving. We all experience ourselves through these basic sensory channels, and they are the entryways to your inner process.

The following basic awareness exercise serves as a foundation for following and working with others in deeply internal states, and it helps you learn to follow your own inner process. These methods can be used cross-culturally, even if you do not understand the person's language. It seems that people around the world have common forms of sensory awareness.

Instructions (*in pairs with one person leading you through the steps, or alone with one person leading the whole group through the exercise, taking time and pausing after each step; 10 to 15 minutes*)

1. **Sit quietly.** Find a sitting position that is comfortable. Just sit for a few moments quietly.

2. **Bring your attention to your breathing.** Notice the rhythm of your breathing; notice whether your breath is shallow or deep, held or fluid, regular or irregular. Just notice your own style of breathing. Do not try to change it consciously; just notice it.

3. **Ask about sensory channels.** When you begin to focus on your inner experience, you will notice that you are hearing things (audition) such as sounds or inner dialogue, seeing things (visual), feeling things in your body (proprioception), or making small movements (kinesthesia), or experiencing some combination of these.

   Now, if you are seeing, then look. If you are hearing, then listen. If you are feeling, then feel. If you are moving, then move.

4. **Amplify.** Now, amplify or strengthen the experience in the channel in which it is occurring.

   For example, if you notice that you are seeing an image, look even more closely at that image. Notice all the details, see the exact colors, notice the forms. You can also try to make the image even larger or, as an alternative, zoom in and look at one part of that image in great detail.

   If you are hearing a sound, listen to it more intensely or make it louder. If it is a voice, try to find out if it is a male or a female voice. How old is the being that is speaking?

   If you are moving, notice exactly how you are moving. Where does the movement begin? Amplify the quality (light, strong, quick, or the like) and direction of the movement (upward, downward, to the side, toward or away from you, on the diagonal), and make the movement a bit larger. Use other body parts to move in the same way.

5. **Switch channels.** If you are feeling something, focus on this feeling. Notice where the feeling originates. Notice the type of feeling you are

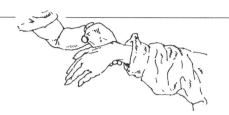

experiencing, such as pressure, sharpness, coldness, weakness, pounding. Feel this a bit more, and let this feeling spread just a bit to more parts of the body. Now switch channels to broaden and unfold your experience by filling it out and giving it even greater expression. If you are hearing something, try to make a movement that goes along with that sound. For example, if you are hearing a loud voice, make large or intense motions that mirror the strength and quality of that sound.

If you are feeling something, perhaps you can make a picture of that feeling. A firm pressure in your head might be imaged as a vise that is closing in on a piece of wood, holding it steady.

If you are moving, try to feel that movement in your body. For example, if one of your hands is lightly moving upward, feel this experience of lightness in your whole body.

6. **Let your experience unfold in various channels.** Allow the experience to express itself in all of these channels and to unfold naturally. Give it room to express itself in great depth and color.

For example, if your hand is lightly moving upward, amplify this by moving your whole body in this way. Now add other channels. Make an image of this light feeling. Perhaps you will see clouds rising. Begin to make sounds that mirror this light feeling, and feel this lightness in your whole body.

Continue following your experience in any way it would like to express itself.

7. **Discuss.** After 10 minutes, share your inner experiences with someone else.

Inner Work Basics

Quick Review

1. Sit quietly.
2. Bring your attention to your breathing.
3. Ask about sensory channels.
4. Amplify.
5. Switch channels.
6. Let your experience unfold in various channels.
7. Discuss.

Summary of Learning from Chapter 7

❖ Think about why you want to do this kind of work.

❖ Experiment with your internal states to find out what it is like to be in a deep trance or coma.

❖ Learn as much as you can about your own altered states and important altered-state experiences you have had in your life.

❖ Explore the meaning of your own life and what you would do if you had six months to live.

❖ Become acquainted with your views about death, dying, and an afterlife.

❖ Remember times when you have been afraid of dying. Use this fear to learn about aspects of yourself that want to "die" and parts that want to emerge into life.

❖ Learn to follow and deepen your own inner states by noticing, amplifying, and unfolding experiences in their sensory channels.

Note

1. See Arnold Mindell's *Working on Yourself Alone* for more information and exercises on working on yourself alone.

Observation, Signals, and Communication

C hapters 8 and 9 present rudimentary coma exercises. These exercises provide the most fundamental skills, laying the groundwork for all other exercises that follow. The exercises progress step by step and expand on one another. All exercises are geared toward learning to adapt to and join the communication system of the comatose person, not expecting the person to relate to us in ordinary ways we are accustomed to. You are letting the comatose person know you are present by joining and responding lovingly to his altered state. In essence, you are saying, "I am here with you, and I am going to join you where you are and assist you in following your inner experiences." This metaskill allows the comatose person to attend to and value his inner processes, knowing that someone is there as a loving companion.

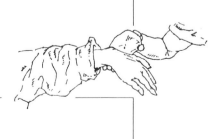

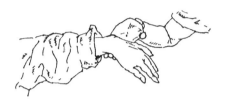

Learn from Each Other

In these exercises, as well as all other exercises in this manual, the person acting as if she were in a coma should not only be the recipient of interventions. She should also remain aware enough to be able to give constructive feedback to her partner during, and especially after, the exercises. This kind of feedback is the best way to help one another learn. The comatose person is an assistant in learning.

After each exercise, the person in the "coma" should try to answer the following questions:

❖ What did your partner do that was helpful?

❖ What was less useful?

❖ What would have been even more helpful to you?

Exercise 1

Gathering Pertinent Information

If you were to receive a phone call from someone telling you that a relative is in a coma—or if you are on site near the person for the first time—what information would be important to gain in order to familiarize yourself as much as possible with the overall situation? To be of as much assistance as possible to family, friends, and the comatose individual, what questions would you ask?

Instructions (*in pairs, 15 minutes; then 20-minute discussion with the whole group*)

1. **Choose questions.** What questions would be important for you to ask during your first phone call or visit?

2. **Articulate why the questions are important.** Why did you select those particular questions? What information and responses are you looking for? Why?

3. **Write down questions.** Write down these questions now.

4. **Take another look.** Take another look at your questions and ask yourself, "Did I consider…" [the following]:

❖ The family?

❖ The person's overall medical situation?

❖ The origins of the coma?

❖ The comatose person's momentary behavior?

❖ The state the person was in before she went into the coma?

5. **Discuss answers with the group, and turn to Chapter 3.** Discuss your responses to steps 1 through 4 with the whole group; then turn to Chapter 3 and talk together about the list of questions and the discussion following those questions.

Gathering Pertinent Information

Quick Review

1. **Choose questions.**
2. **Articulate why the questions are important.**
3. **Write down questions.**
4. **Take another look.**
5. **Discuss answers with the group, and turn to Chapter 3.**

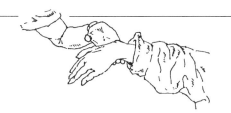

Exercise 2

Foundations of Communication

Typically, someone working with a comatose person for the first time relates to that person as if he were in a normal state of consciousness, such as by saying, "Hello, how are you today?" Yet people in comatose states experience and express themselves differently than they expressed themselves before the coma.

The comatose person is not talking or giving ordinary verbal feedback that we are accustomed to and is most likely going through different types of experiences than he did in normal consciousness. He may be making unusual motions or sounds. Therefore coma work requires that we learn new ways of communicating.

Coma is a call for a special kind of relationship—one that is specifically tailored to the state of consciousness the person is in. Discuss the following issues with a partner or with your whole group.

Instructions *(in pairs, 5 minutes per person; then possible group discussion)*

1. **Discuss communication styles.** How do you think you should relate to someone who is in a deeply internal state? Typical responses include the following:

❖ Sensitively.

❖ With touch.

❖ With meditation.

2. **Think about yourself.** How would you like to be related to if you were in this state? Typical responses include the following:

❖ With compassion.

❖ Knowing that the person cares about me.

❖ Knowing that the helper wants to relate to me and not make me relate to her.

❖ Helping me follow my inner states.

3. **Review notes.** Now take some time with your partner or the whole group to review "First Steps" about coma work for family and friends at the beginning of Chapter 4 as a preparation for the upcoming exercises.

Foundations of Communication

Quick Review

1. **Discuss communication styles.**
2. **Think about yourself.**
3. **Review notes.**

One of the best ways to learn new methods of communication is to free yourself from having to do things right. In the beginning of your learning, you should have the liberty to try all kinds of methods and even make mistakes! The following experience is designed to allow you to freely experiment with many forms of communication.

Exercise 3

Experimenting with Communication

In this exercise one person is the coma helper. The other person should lie down and act as though she were in a deep trance or comatose state. Experiment with all the communication styles you can think of (such as touch, movement, or sound) while respecting the person with whom you are working. I have seen some of my students begin to sing; others have reclined next to the person and tried to get into the same state as the "comatose" person, and still others have used their noses to touch the person's feet!

After the exercise, the person who was pretending to be comatose should give feedback to the helper about her experience of the helper's various communication styles.

Instructions (*in pairs; 10 minutes per person*)

1. **Get permission.** Ask your partner if you can experiment with different methods of communicating. Find out if there are any things that you should not do, such as making sudden sounds or touching certain areas of the body. Then, if your partner agrees, she should lie down and act as if she were in a comatose state.

2. **Experiment with different forms of communication.** Try various ways of communicating, such as talking, singing, touching, moving the person, and so forth. Be respectful, yet experimental. Don't worry about "getting it right." Enjoy the freedom to be creative.

3. **Ask for feedback.** After five minutes or so, ask your partner to give you feedback using the following questions as a springboard.

❖ How was your partner affected by the various communication methods you used?

❖ Which communication methods seemed helpful, which disturbing? Why?

❖ Which methods would your partner have liked the most?

Experimenting with Communication

Quick Review

1. **Get permission.**
2. **Experiment with different forms of communication.**
3. **Ask for feedback.**

Exercise 4

Observation of Minimal Signals

A process-oriented approach to comatose states considers all signals, that is, bits of communication, as potentially meaningful, even if they are autonomic. There is a hidden world of communication occurring in even the most minimal signals, such as twitches of the lips, shaking of a finger, or changes in coloration of the skin.

Minimal signals are the gateways to interaction, to dreams and inner experiences. In a comatose person, we have seen tiny signals of the mouth unfold into the expression of deep feelings, minimal movements of the hand into a warm embrace, slight sounds into a song.

It is difficult to notice minimal signals because many of us have learned that it is impolite to notice the gestures of others. The following exercise is meant to reawaken your senses to the multitude of tiny signals that you might notice from a comatose person.

The kinds of expressions and movements that a comatose person makes are organized by her altered-state experiences and current physical limitations and may be very different than we had previously imagined. Therefore it is most helpful to practice speaking in sensory-grounded, neutral terms that heighten the comatose person's awareness of her individual experiences without interpreting these signals. Later, we will experiment with bringing in fantasies or intuitions and communicating with aspects of body communication through feeling, sound, touch, and movement.

Instructions *(15 minutes, all together as a group)*

1. **One person lies down on the floor.** One person should lie on the floor and act as if she were in a comatose state.

2. **Observe.** The others should observe the "comatose" person. Notice any subtle signals (such as breathing patterns, breathing changes, sounds, and minimal movements of the face, eyes, mouth, and cheeks).

3. **Describe signals.** Everyone should describe aloud the signals they observe in sensory-grounded terms.

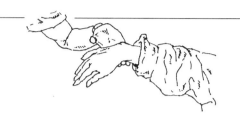

Once again, *sensory-grounded* refers to the senses. When we describe phenomena in sensory-grounded terms, it means that we state exactly what we notice in terms of the senses, that is, in terms of movement, sound, feeling, or visualization, without interpreting those observations. For example:

❖ The head is turned slightly to the right.

❖ The mouth is puckered.

❖ The hands are curled inward slightly.

❖ There is a red patch on the left side of the face.

❖ The rhythm of the breath is alternately slow and then fast.

❖ The person makes quiet sounds during each exhalation.

Check to make sure that you are not interpreting but simply describing exactly the signals you notice.

Sensory-grounded descriptions avoid the danger of misinterpreting what a person is experiencing. All of us have a tendency to interpret what we observe, imagining what someone else is experiencing. We see facial expressions and imagine pain or sadness. Be careful. Our interpretations are based on our familiarity with these expressions as we know them in ordinary life, not on their emergence from an altered-state experience. Statements students typically make that are not sensory grounded include the following:

❖ She looks sad.

❖ The lips show anger.

❖ She is getting nervous.

Attending to minimal signals is an awesome experience. You know what it is like to be attended to with such care. It is a special experience when someone sensitively notices your subtle expressions and signals. It makes you feel seen and supported and brings you added awareness and appreciation of your own inner process. As a coma worker, when you notice signals, you heighten the comatose person's awareness of her own communications and thereby enable her to follow and unfold her inner experiences.

4. **Observe again.** After a few minutes, start over. Observe and describe signals again. This time, use the attitude of appreciating everything, that is, not taking anything for granted. That means appreciating even the smallest, seemingly insignificant signals. With this feeling in mind, you will begin to notice signals you might ordinarily overlook. Observe the person who is lying down again. If you do not take anything for granted, what signals do you now observe that you did not notice before? Describe these in sensory-grounded terms.

5. **Look for signals you may have missed.** In case you didn't notice the following signals, go back and observe again.

❖ Position of body parts: direction and position of the arms, elbows, hands, legs, knees, chest, and head. Are the feet together or separate? Are the elbows close to the body or further out?

❖ Overall body posture, such as lying with the body flat, with the legs pulled up, with hands on the stomach, with the upper body turned slightly to the side.

❖ Direction the hair has fallen.

❖ Breathing rate.

❖ Changes in breathing.

❖ Whether breathing seems to originate in the upper chest or solar plexus.

❖ Holding of the breath.

❖ Variations in color of skin in different parts of the face.

❖ Eyelids open or closed. If closed, is there fluttering? Can you see the eyes moving? If open, do the eyes stare? Do the pupils dilate?

❖ Smells.

❖ Mouth and facial expressions, signs of tension or relaxation.

❖ Is the head centered, slightly tilting backward?

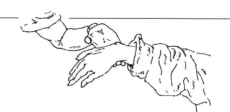

- ❖ Is the chin jutting up a bit or pressed down?
- ❖ Muscles of the limbs: signs of tension, relaxation, shaking.
- ❖ Position of the legs.
- ❖ Position of feet and toes.
- ❖ Sounds associated with breathing?
- ❖ Minimal movements.
- ❖ Swallowing.
- ❖ Position of the hands: are the hands doing the same thing? Are the hands or one hand out to the side away from the body, on the stomach, on the chest, on the pelvis? Are they turned outward, inward, or in fists?
- ❖ What are the fingers doing, especially the thumbs?

6. **Try exercise with another person.** Now repeat instructions 1 through 4 with another person lying down.

Observation of Minimal Signals

Quick Review

1. **One person lies on the floor.**
2. **Observe.**
3. **Describe signals.**
4. **Observe again.**
5. **Look for signals you may have missed.**
6. **Try with another person.**

Exercise 5

Joining through the Breath

You may have noticed in the last exercise that the kinds of signals we observe belong to the most fundamental ways we communicate—through the breath, the use of our eyes, sounds, and movements. We assist a comatose person by noticing and joining these basic methods of communication.

Let's begin by focusing on the breath. Breathing is one of the strongest signals to follow when working with someone in a coma. You will need to notice the rhythm of the breath, the depth, and sound.

One of the most powerful ways to get in contact with someone in a coma is to pace the rhythm of the person's breathing. When you do this, the comatose person feels your presence and that you are joining him in his process and pace of communication.

In this exercise, you will come very close to your partner and gently speak to and touch him in cadence with this breathing rate. Know that the best communication occurs when your nonverbal communication (touch) also mirrors the pace of your speech.

As you get close to your partner and mirror his rate of breathing, use your sensitivity to feel into and align yourself with the person's state.

Instructions (*approximately 15 minutes per person; 5 to 10 minutes to practice, 5 minutes to discuss*)

1. **Read notes and try the exercise.** Read the notes below and then turn to Chapter 4, Exercise 1, and try steps 1 through 6 and step 8 in pairs.

❖ **Tuning in sentiently.** Before you approach the "comatose" person, take your time and try to tune in and sense where the person is. Arny and I use the term *sentience*[1] to describe a deep, feeling, preverbal state of consciousness in which you *feel* your way into the person's altered state. It is an inner meditative state of awareness in which you have the sense of intimately joining the comatose person in his world rather than feeling like an outsider who is in a different state of consciousness. (See the discussion of metaskills on page 152 for more on sentience.) Sentience is

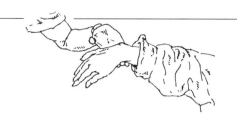

very difficult to describe in words because it is a preverbal type of feeling, which occurs before the feeling is expressed in words. I assume that most of us know this type of feeling if we are interested in this work. In the exercise, try to adjust and feel your way, sentiently, into the rhythm and pace of the person's breathing.

❖ **On getting close.** When you try this exercise, sit close to your partner and put your head as near to his ear as feels comfortable (Figure 1, page 67). You do not have to look straight at the person as if you were studying him, although you will try to notice any signals the person makes. It is hard to describe how to do this. Look but don't look. Feel your way into the person's altered state. Perhaps put your head slightly to the side or down, or gaze in a non-intrusive way as you sentiently join the person's inner world.

If you experience shyness in being so close, it may be helpful to know that all people in coma we have worked with seem to greatly appreciate the physical closeness of the caregiver's sensitive voice and presence near theirs. Even a person who has been quite shy before going into a coma, when approached and communicated with in a loving and sensitive way, seems to value this intimacy of contact. Remember that people in this state are very isolated and appreciate loving contact. We will address the helper's intimacy and contact issues in Chapter 10.

❖ **Speaking on the exhalation.** One of the most effective ways of speaking to someone in a coma is to speak gently in the rhythm of his breathing. That is, speak when the person exhales, and pause during the inhale. Then speak again during the exhale. This mirrors the way we all speak, which is only during exhalation. Speak in a warm, sensitive tone of voice.

❖ **Touching the wrist**. To enhance your communication, touch the person in rhythm with the breath. We suggest touching the wrist because it is an extremity and therefore touching it is a gentler, less intrusive way to initiate contact. (As an alternative, you can do the same thing with the elbow if the person's hand and wrist are resting on the body.)

Hold the wrist, pressing gently on the inhalation and relaxing this pressure on the exhalation (see Figure 2, page 68). Pressing during inhalation mirrors the tension of the muscles of the lungs during inhalation. When you release your pressure, you mirror the relaxation in the muscles during exhalation.

Before you touch someone, it is important that you tell the person you are going to do so, and where. Touching someone is an immense project that requires great care. After you have become acquainted with the person and worked for some time, however, you will not have to continue mentioning everything you are doing.

❖ **On belief.** In this exercise you encourage the person to experiment with believing in and following whatever is happening inside of him. Sometimes deep trances persist, apart from medical difficulties, because the person resists or is shy about his inner experiences. Or trances may persist because people on the outside do not value the comatose person's inner experiences.

Asking the comatose person to experiment with believing in the experiences he is having means that he has permission to trust in his inner experiences. He knows that you are there supporting and appreciating these experiences as well.

2. **Discuss.** Share your experiences with your partner.

3. **Try with others.** At another point, try the same exercise with more than one coma helper, coordinating your work with other parts of the body, as explained in Chapter 4, Exercise 1 (step 7).

Joining through the Breath
Quick Review
1. Read the notes and try the exercise.
2. Discuss.
3. Try with others.

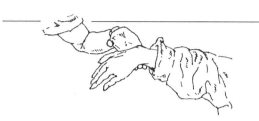

Exercise 6

Minimal Cues and Channels

We now extend the preceding exercise by adding sensory channels in which the person may be experiencing her process. Once again, we are going to the most basic level of experience: the way our experiences express themselves through the various sensory modalities.

Use this exercise to help the "comatose" person follow herself, and as an experiment in which you will guess which sensory channel your partner is experiencing. Afterwards, get feedback from your partner about your guesses.

Instructions *(in pairs; 15 minutes per person)*

1. **Approach.** One person lies down and imagines being in a deep trance state. The partner begins with following the breath as in the previous exercise. After a couple of minutes, encourage the "comatose" person to follow her inner experiences. Say something like the following in the rhythm of her breath:

   *"All you have to do *… is follow what is happening inside of you *…that will show us the way."*

   Note: Asterisks with ellipses represent pauses paralleling inhalation.

2. **Mention sensory channels, and respond to feedback.** Speaking in the rhythm of her breath, tell the person:

   *"You might be **feeling** things *(pause)…you might be **seeing** things *… or **hearing** things *…or maybe you are making **movements**…* If you are **feeling** something, then **feel** it *…if you are **seeing** something, then **look** at it *…if you are **hearing** something, then **listen** *…if you are **moving**, then follow these **movements**."*

   Pause a bit as you mention each channel, watching for feedback. Notice where you get the strongest response, and encourage the person to follow her experiences. A big breath may indicate a response to a particular channel. When you see a response, say something like:

"Oh yes, feeling... hmmm." Or *"Oooh, that was a big breath, humm, seeing something..."*

A strong response could be encouraged by talking about seeing in a general way, without mentioning anything in particular:

"Oh, seeing...yes, I see that, too...amazing, looking...Yes, seeing, look, watch..."

Or, with other sensory channels:

"Listening, hmmm, sounds, hearing, just listen..."

"Feeling, yes, sensations, feel what you are feeling..."

"Yes, little movements, hmmm, moving."

If you are unsure about which channel the person is experiencing herself in, just encourage her in a general way to follow whatever she is seeing, hearing, feeling, or any small movements that arise.

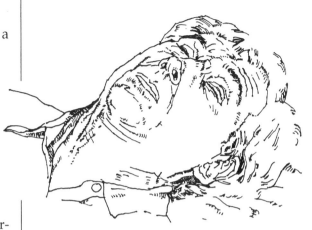

Fig. 50
Trying to focus

3. **Link signals to channels, and comment about them.** You can also guess the sensory channel by noticing specific signals. Here are some typical signals and the sensory-oriented channels with which they are associated.

   Just before people focus on something, their *upper lip* and *nose* scrunch down a bit. The muscles between the eyes contract and form a crevice (Figure 50). The person is trying to see something.

   Also, when the person is just about to begin to focus visually on something, you might notice a slight twitch of the *eyebrows* as they slightly come together. Or this may occur only with one eyebrow if the person is in a coma associated with a narcotic overdose, a stroke, or other organic problems. One eyebrow moving up by itself could be a sign of concentration on something in particular.

   Swallowing is one of the most common signals. Although swallowing is a reflex, the moment when someone swallows is most often an indication of thinking a thought and is typically related to feeling. Although

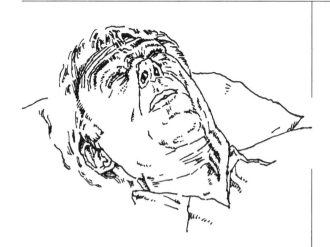

Fig. 51
Muscular contraction in
jaw indicating feeling

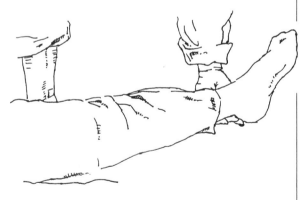

Fig. 52
Stiffness in legs

we are not sure which channel the thought is occurring in, it is helpful to say:

"Oh, a thought, that's an important thought. Believe in the feelings and thoughts you're having."

Muscular contractions in the *lower jaw* frequently signal a feeling response (Figure 51). Acknowledge what you are seeing:

"I see a quiver there, maybe you are feeling something."

A typical signal you will see from people who have suffered from brain injury is decorticate posturing. The hand or hands are stiffly pulled up toward the chest, fingers pointed toward the heart, crooked in, and slightly jittering. With decerebrate posturing, the hands are turned outward and crooked in an upward direction and there is tension in the arms (Figures 29 and 30, page 90). The legs also tend to display decorticate or decerebrate posturing and can be very stiff (Figure 52). These are types of movement signals. Other movement signals include jittering of the hands or arms, twitches of the face, and so forth.

Eye movements to the left or right, whether the eye is opened or closed, frequently indicate that the person is listening to something (Figure 53). Say something that encourages the person to listen. If a person looks up intently, this most often means seeing something. Sometimes the head also tilts back slightly. If the eyes remain glazed and open, the person may not be looking but may be hearing or feeling something.

A fluttering of the eyelids when the eyes are closed almost always signals deep inner feeling. Encourage the person to feel whatever she is experiencing.

4. **Comment on channels.** Again, mention the channel you think the comatose person is experiencing. Here are some additional methods of responding.

❖ If you think she is seeing something, encourage her by saying in a neutral, non-interpretative way:

"Look at that! I see it, too! Wow!... Looking."

❖ If there are slight movements you might say:

"Yes, movement, oh those motions, they are important. Movement is happening, I wonder where it will go… Sometimes movements go up and sometimes they go down."

❖ If the person's eyes flutter, you could say:

"Oh, a deep breath! Wow! Feeling something."

❖ If the person's eyes move sideways toward one ear, you might reinforce listening closely:

"Listening, sound, hmmmm, just listen…"

5. **Watch for feedback.** Notice whether you receive a particularly good response to your comments about channels from the person lying down. If so, continue using sounds and words to deepen your communication. Continue to encourage the person to follow her awareness of whatever is happening.

If you do not receive feedback, then try another channel or simply encourage the person to follow her experiences, whether they involve visual, auditory, feeling, or movement sensations.

On channel changing. If you are working with people in many degrees of coma and wakefulness, it is helpful to know how to change channels, as described in Chapter 7. Here is a story to illustrate changing channels. After an operation for a brain tumor, a woman was flailing around in her bed. She had IV lines in her arms, and it was dangerous for her to move so much. Arny encouraged her to make a channel change from movement to visualization. He said, "Go for it. Don't sit up, but do it in your imagination and get what you need." At that point the woman swallowed. "Feel it," he said. Finally, it became apparent that she wanted water. She was thirsty.

6. **Discuss.** After ten minutes or so, ask your partner to sit up and discuss the exercise with one another. Compare your channel guesses to the "comatose" person's actual experience. Learn from each other in this way about signals and sensory channels.

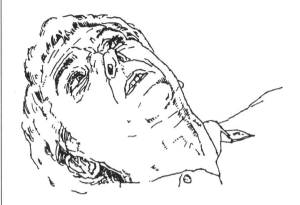

Fig. 53
Eyes to left or right,
indicating listening

Minimal Cues and Channels
Quick Review
1. **Approach.**
2. **Mention sensory channels, and respond to feedback.**
3. **Link signals to channels, and comment.**
4. **Comment on channels.**
5. **Watch for feedback.**
6. **Discuss.**

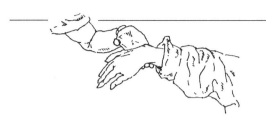

Exercise 7

Identifying and Deepening Your Metaskills

Feeling qualities, or metaskills[2], form the essential foundation of all these skills. They communicate your special form of presence to the person in coma and create an intimate, loving setting. The way you feel is crucial to your effectiveness in communicating with the comatose person.

Perhaps you have had these metaskills from birth. Or, perhaps, mentioning them will bring them to birth in you. You may exude these qualities without identifying them. Many of us are involved in this work because we are connected to these deep, feeling qualities.

Instructions (*10 minutes per person, or all together as a group*)

1. **Identify important metaskills.** What metaskills do you feel are important in coma work? Possible responses include kindness, sensitivity, love, an appreciation of altered states, companionship, curiosity, and openness.

2. **Identify your metaskills.** What feeling qualities that are helpful do you bring naturally to this work?

3. **Consider basic metaskills.** Some of the many metaskills that are helpful in coma work are the following, although they are difficult to describe in words.

One of the deepest metaskills is a sense of *love* and connection to the person with whom you are working. The closer you are to a sense of deep love inside yourself, the more effective your work will be. This loving awareness tells us that although all of us go through separate lives and struggles, and may never have met, we are also all a part of humanity and in some way know one another. It is the deep feeling that everyone is somehow a part of your family. When this attitude pervades your heart and mind, you will draw close to people in coma quickly and in a deep way.

Another metaskill is *openness* or *compassion*. This is a special feeling of respect and compassion for the awesomeness of each individual's unique process. This feeling opens us up to embracing the multitude of ways in which we express ourselves, in ordinary as well as altered states of consciousness.

As mentioned earlier, a metaskill that I call *taking nothing for granted* allows you to appreciate the most minimal of signals (signals we normally ignore) and to cherish them as entryways to deep experiences. This metaskill requires both a scientific attitude with which we notice signals and a feeling quality of compassion that embraces them.

A very important metaskill is *patience*. When working with people in coma, particularly coma resulting from brain injury, the recuperation period may take a long time. A great amount of inner processing and re-education stands between the comatose state and everyday reality, so coma workers need an abundance of patience to allow the person's experiences to unfold at their own unique pace.

When you get to know your own altered states and live more closely to your sense of life and death, you develop a metaskill we call *"I've been there, too."* You have the sense that you are not really that different from the comatose person. You know somehow where the person is and can join her rather than feeling like an outsider who is simply a "helper." You are a true companion instead of an observer.

When you do this, you develop the metaskill of *sentience*. When you are sentient, you are in a deep feeling state in which you are connected with the comatose person in a deep way, on a level that is preverbal, before you can even speak about it.

Many people interested in coma work are very sentient. They seem to sense and feel things even before they can say them. They can "tune in" to where someone is. Everyone knows this sense when you listen to a beautiful piece of music or see a beautiful dance. You feel something deeply but may not be able to formulate what moves you in exact words.

A sentient coma worker climbs into the comatose person's world, even without speaking. She looks natural and seems to be totally at home

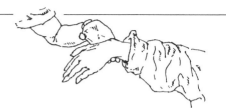

with the comatose person. She does not look at the person as an outside object but seamlessly joins in the process that is unfolding.

When you encourage a comatose person to believe in her inner experiences, you are, in essence, encouraging the person to follow and trust her own inner sentient tendencies as the path to unfolding her inner world, even if she does not yet know exactly what they are or where they are heading.

This sentient metaskill connects to another metaskill: a *beginner's mind*. Here you are open to and believe in experiences even if you do not understand them completely and do not necessarily know their origins. You are present for this unknown sentient world and try to follow nature as well as possible.

4. **Take notes.** Write down your thoughts on metaskills in your personal log.

*Identifying and Deepening
Your Metaskills*

Quick Review

1. **Identify important metaskills.**
2. **Identify your metaskills.**
3. **Consider basic metaskills.**
4. **Take notes.**

Exercise 8

Responding to Signals and Adding Sound

In this exercise, we not only follow the breath but also attend to each signal the comatose person makes. Appreciating even the most minimal signals is very important; these expressions are the beginning of communication and indicate the presence of inner experiences.

For example, irregular breathing may indicate that the person is in the middle of a strong experience and changes are happening internally. If the head and arms are moving all at once, this usually indicates that there is a lot of expression which is very close to awareness trying to happen. By measuring the pulse you can ascertain whether the person is becoming more peaceful or more excited. (The pulse rate usually increases when someone is excited and may decrease when the person is resting or at peace, although the heart rate may also increase as a result of such factors as a rising temperature or lowered blood volume.)

The comatose person feels related to and accompanied if you notice and respond through sound and touch to all of his communications, no matter how small they may be. (You may discover that you feel shy about making sounds. Don't worry. We will focus on your shyness more deeply in Chapter 10.)

Instructions *(in pairs, 15 minutes per person; 10 minutes for practice and 5 minutes for feedback)*

1. **Consider possible responses.** In this exercise you will use verbal responses to let the person know that you have noticed his signals. You can say, for example, in a loving, affirmative way:

"Yes, I see your lips moving. When you do that, I know you are there."

"I feel your fingers squeezing, hmmm, yes!"

"Wow, a big breath. It's a pleasure to be with you here."

You can also use your voice to make blank sounds—we call this *blank accessing*—to let the comatose person know that you have noticed her signals. The most effective vocal responses are made in an encouraging

After you try this exercise, read the two examples that follow, which demonstrate this method. I hope that these will give you a greater sense of the flow of the work and also provide a sense of subtle and crucial elements of this work that are difficult to describe.

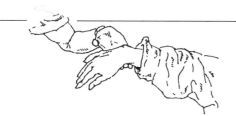

tone and mirror the quality, strength, and rhythm of the comatose person's signals. Remember, do not interpret what you notice: simply respond in an open, encouraging manner.

The following kinds of sounds are suggested as mirroring particular signals:

- Twitches and spasms: staccato-like sounds (such as *"Eh—ah—eh"*).

- Sleepy, gentle, and quiet motions: coddling, mothering sounds, quiet and soothing (such as *"Mmmmm ... ooohh ... yessss ..."*).

- Tugging and fighting motions: intense, louder, struggling, and encouraging sounds (such as *"Whoa! Yeah! Wow!"*).

Adding sounds. Once you begin to make sounds with someone, you can start a communication system by adding to the sounds that you make.

Imagine that the person makes the sound *"ahhh"* and you respond likewise with *"ahhh."*

After a while, add something to your sound, such as *"ahhhh-ah-ha!"* and notice what kind of feedback you receive. If you do not get any feedback, try another sound add-on with a slightly different intonation. If the comatose person responds with more sounds, you have started a communication system and can experiment back and forth with this new language.

You can do this with words as well. If the comatose person says a particular word or seems to respond to a word you have used, say the word again, stressing different parts of it. Try different intonations. For example, if the person responds to the word *life*, experiment with repeating the word a number of times, each time stressing a different part of the word, such as:

"LLLLLLLife!"

or

"LIIIIve"

or

Note: Most of us have the natural tendency to relate in a very quiet manner when someone is in a coma. This is especially important when you first approach the person. However, if the person's signals are more intense and energetic, it is most helpful to communicate in like manner, that is, with more expressive responses. In other words, use the same intensity, volume and energy in your sounds as the sounds and signals of the comatose person.

"LiVING"

or continue to amplify the word, such as:

"Life! Living! Wow, amazing, life ...!!!"

In this exercise you notice any moments when you receive the most feedback from the comatose person and continue to interact creatively.

2. **Try the exercise.** Turn to Chapter 4, Exercise 3, and try this method.

3. **Discuss.** After the exercise, discuss the following questions with your partner:

❖ Did you feel comfortable responding to various signals with words and sound?

❖ Were you able to mirror these signals in rhythm and intensity?

❖ How did you feel when you were adding on sounds?

Examples

Attending to Minimal Signals

Recently, Arny and I gave coma assistance over the telephone to Mark, a man who was in another city with Sue, a cousin of his who was in a coma. Sue had had a stroke and had been without oxygen for an unknown period of time. The medical staff was uncertain regarding the extent of brain injury. Mark was on site, at Sue's bedside, when he phoned us.

> We first asked Mark which side of the bed he was on. He told us that he was on the right side. We told Mark to put his mouth and face near Sue and then speak gently into her left ear and say, *"Sue, this is me, Mark, I'm here."*
>
> Mark tried this and said that Sue made some small motions with her legs. We told Mark to say, *"Sue, when you move around, I know you're here."* [Mark repeated this.] We then told him to repeat the following: *"I'm going to trust what's inside of you as the path."* We told Mark, "Watch the facial expressions Sue makes and see if anything moves at all."

Responding to Signals and Adding Sound

Quick Review

1. **Consider possible responses.**
2. **Try the exercise.**
3. **Discuss.**

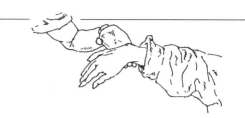

Mark noticed that Sue's eyes moved and her mouth moved slightly as well. We suggested that he say to her, *"I saw your eyes flicker a bit and your mouth move. That shows you're here, too!"*

Mark repeated this and then said that Sue made a slight motion with her head. We told Mark to say, *"I saw your head move, that's very important to me."* We continued, encouraging Mark to speak slowly and in rhythm with Sue's breath, *"I'm with you, I love you, I'm Mark."*

We then said to Mark, "Take her left wrist in your hand and each time she breathes in, squeeze it, and say, *"I'm here"* and watch if there is any feedback at all." We encouraged him to say, *"Sue, I know you're here, it's wonderful to feel you."*

Mark said that Sue's mouth moved again. We told him to put one of his fingers on her mouth and say, *"Wonderful to see your mouth move!"* Then her legs began to move and we encouraged him to say in an excited tone, *"Wonderful! Your mouth is moving and your legs!"*

We had to get off the phone, but we encouraged Mark to continue by himself, making an excited response every time he noticed a signal from Sue—something like, *"Oh, your beautiful eyebrow has moved! It's me, Mark, and it's you there!"*

Making loving, affirmative comments about the comatose person's signals helps the person become aware of and use her body signals to communicate.

A Supervision Session

Here is another example of a supervision session. Two therapists were with a comatose person. They initially felt that it was quite hard to establish communication with the comatose woman and that there was not much response. You will see how sensitive shifts in their communication methods elicit a great deal of communication from the comatose person. You will also notice the fluctuation between a sleepy state and a more wakeful state and how to follow the flow of both.[3]

In this example, Arny is giving moment-to-moment feedback on the telephone to Jean, one of the coma helpers. The feeling quality of the interaction is of utmost importance.

> Jean tells Arny that the comatose woman is lying on her side. The woman's eyes are open, and she is breathing quietly. Arny instructs Jean to speak in a warm, rhythmic, slow, and loving tone of voice.
>
> Arny: [To Jean] Is she lying down?
>
> Jean: Yes.
>
> Arny: Put the phone in one of your ears, Jean, so you can listen to me. Bend down and get close to her with your other ear. [Jean does this, bending down low, close to the woman's face.]
>
> Arny: How close are you?
>
> Jean: About a half a hand away. Oh, she made a big movement!
>
> Arny: Breathe in the rate of her breathing. Yes, that's it... Put your face as close to hers as you dare, even closer, touch her cheek with yours, if you want. Have you ever been this close to her?
>
> Jean: No, not really.
>
> Arny: Tell Mike [the other coma helper] to put his hands on her feet, pressing in conjunction with her breathing.
>
> Jean: She made a big sigh and swallowed.
>
> Arny: Yes, breathe with her and mumble sounds that go with the breath. [Jean does this by making "oohing" sounds corresponding to the woman's breathing rhythm.]
>
> Jean: Oh. [Now talking to the woman and simultaneously to Arny on the phone, Jean comments about the woman's signals.] *"Your eyes go up and down, and some mouth movements happen!"*
>
> Arny: Put your hands on her chin, if you feel comfortable, and see if she reacts to that.
>
> Jean: *Yes … your legs are pushing … whoops … and now your eyes are going down …*
>
> Arny: [Arny tells Jean to repeat what he says to the comatose woman. He talks slowly, almost sleepily, and warmly.] *"Good*

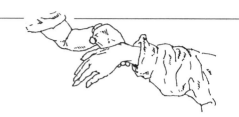

night … it's very nice … to take a pause …" [He tells Jean to stroke her head.]

Jean: [Commenting about the woman's signals] *Ooh, you make movements when we touch you.*

Arny: [Tells Jean to say] *"Yes, wonderful…wonderful to be with you here …"*

Jean: *Yes and eyes going slowly down …*

Arny: Sing a little song to her, Jean, like *"dum di dum di dum, row, row, row your boat …"*

Jean: [Sings slowly and sweetly and then] *Oooh, your eyes opened!*

Arny: [Telling Jean to repeat] *"What nice eyes!"*

Jean: *Beautiful eyes. And now your eyes close.*

Arny: [Slowly and rhythmically, he tells Jean to repeat] *"Once they open and once they close. How exciting! And what a pleasure to be here with you my friend …"*

Jean: *Eyes open again. Hello there!*

Arny: *"Good morning …oooh, yeah …"*

Jean: *Yes, that's nice, your eyes close again.*

Arny: *"Sleep, sleep as long as you need. I'm here."*

Jean: [To Arny] Another big movement.

Arny: [A bit louder] *"Woah, but wake up when you like. Yes, movement!"*

Jean: *Yes, you are opening your eyes and looking almost right at me. How lovely.*

Arny: *"Good morning, what do you know … you're beautiful …!"*

Notes on Feedback

One of the most important skills of coma work is your ability to notice feedback from the comatose person. If the comatose person begins to respond more to what you are saying or doing, you are on a good track. If you receive no response, then notice other signals, try other techniques, or take a break.

How can you tell positive from negative feedback? This is one of the questions most frequently asked by coma students. One of the basic rules is: no feedback is negative feedback. If you are in a comatose state, the strongest way to give negative feedback is simply by going deeper into the coma and not responding at all. That means a loss or lessening of communication. Of course, the person may also stop communicating simply because he is tired.

Positive feedback is any response in communication to your input. A deep breath is usually positive feedback to something you are doing. Watch for even the tiniest instances of feedback. If the comatose person pulls away when you touch him, don't take it immediately as a sign of not wanting contact. On the contrary, we have seen many such signals turn into wrestling matches and demonstrations of strength. I remember a woman we worked with who had been in a car accident. She had a great deal of tension in her feet and hands. When we pressed up slightly on her hands and the balls of her feet, she pressed back intensely and this was the beginning of a struggle. Through asking her questions (see Chapter 9 on binary communication), she told us she was in the middle of a great battle in which she had to overcome oppressive forces that were putting her down.

A common question about this work is: As a coma worker, can you inadvertently do something that is wrong? If you have a good heart and are sensitive, it is hard to do anything wrong or hurtful. When someone is not able to talk back to give you feedback in the ordinary way, the best thing you can do is have good intentions and sensitively notice and adapt to the person's feedback.

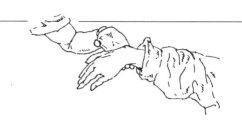

Example of Feedback

The following example of feedback clearly shows the difference in communication that is geared toward the feedback you receive from the comatose person and that which is done with good intention but does not notice feedback.

Friends of a comatose person had heard that snapping fingers and clapping hands loudly in front of the comatose person's face was helpful in bringing someone out of a coma. In this way, the comatose person is supposed to receive strong stimuli which should help awaken the senses and bring the person back to everyday reality.

When we later watched this interaction on videotape, we noticed that the comatose person gave no feedback to the constant clapping, shouting, and snapping of fingers. Instead, he remained staring in one direction and seemed more distant and less accessible.

Then, one of our students began to work with this person, pacing his breathing. The coma helper sat with the man for a while, getting in tune with his breathing rhythm, and gently said that she was there and that he should believe in and follow whatever was happening inside of him.

She sat close and commented lovingly and supportively about the minimal signals that the man made with his mouth and head. As she did this, the man began to respond almost instantaneously, turning his head toward her, leaning slightly to that side, and beginning to make sounds for the first time. This was positive feedback. The sounds continued, and loving "dialogue" developed.

This example shows that what is most helpful are those sensitive interactions that receive the most feedback. The clapping of hands did not elicit any response, whereas pacing the breathing and following minimal cues received positive feedback. When this occurs, there is a tangible feeling that the helper and the comatose person are in intimate communication with one another.

Summary of Learning from Chapter 8

❖ Develop a list of questions to ask when you first learn that someone is comatose. The answers to these questions will give you important information for your work with the comatose person and your interactions with family and medical staff.

❖ Learn new ways of communicating that are adapted to the comatose person's altered state, not to ordinary reality.

❖ Give yourself the permission to experiment freely with many types of communication.

❖ Remember that all communication signals are potentially meaningful. They are the gateways to the comatose person's inner world and doorways to interaction. Appreciate everything, even seemingly insignificant signals.

❖ Speak in the rhythm of the person's breathing rate (as the person exhales), and pace the breathing by pressing the wrist on the inhalation.

❖ Discover the process in the body by following signals and channels. Try to connect the person's signals to sensory-oriented channels.

❖ Respond in a loving, enthusiastic, and sensitive way to the person's signals through the use of sound, words, and touch in order to accompany the comatose person and foster communication.

❖ Try your best not to interpret. Mention exactly what you see by using neutral sensory language.

❖ Remember to watch for feedback and adjust to it. Positive feedback means that you get a response to what you are doing. Negative feedback means no response.

Notes

1. See Arny Mindell's *The Modern Shaman's Guide to the Universe* for a detailed discussion of sentient awareness.
2. *Metaskills* is a word I coined for the feeling attitudes of the therapist or caretaker. See my *Metaskills: The Spiritual Art of Therapy.*
3. See also Chapter 9, Exercise 2, for more on wakeful and sleepy states.

I n this chapter you will learn how to follow a person's body posture, discover inner processes through using movement techniques, and develop methods of asking the comatose person questions that she can answer.

When you are working with someone in a coma there are several ways to discover and come into contact with the person's inner process, including the following:

- Noticing and responding to overt signals you can see, hear, or feel, as we practiced in the last chapter.
- Noticing feedback and responses to your interventions.
- Using your hands, through touch and movement, to access deep inner processes happening in the musculature of the body.
- Using your intuition to imagine into what the comatose person is experiencing.

The following exercises address and deepen the first three methods. We will bring in our intuitions in Chapter 11.

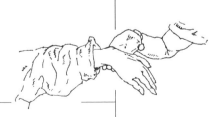

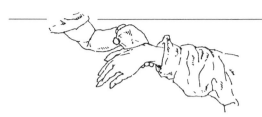

Exercise 1

Basic Postural Awareness

Basic signals from the comatose person, which you can notice and interact with, include common postural, head, arm, and leg signals. The way the person is lying, the position of the body, the hands, and the feet are all signals with potential meaning. Learn to observe, follow, and amplify these signals with the use of your hands.

Instructions (*5 minutes to experiment with postures; 10 minutes per person for the exercise*)

1. **Assume any posture.** Experiment and learn together about posture and signals. One of you should imagine that you are in a coma. Assume any posture that feels natural to you while lying down.

2. **Experiment with amplification.** The coma helper observes and notices posture and positional signals of the "comatose" person. As the helper, you should then experiment with using your hands to amplify the body posture and position. Don't worry if you do not get it right. Give yourself the freedom to experiment, and get feedback from your partner at the end.

To emphasize the significance of postural body signals, including the position and direction of the hands, the head, the feet, tension in the muscles, and so on, here are a few examples from one of my recent coma classes.

One woman lay on the floor with arms stretched upward and fingers slightly extended. Her feet and toes looked slightly outstretched as well. She was imagining flying and hoped her partner would stretch her arms even further upward and her legs further downward. When her partner finally did stretch her arms further upward, the "comatose" woman gave a big breath, indicating positive feedback. Her partner said that she learned to trust such a big breath as an indication of positive feedback—that she was on the right track.

Another class member lay down with his hands gently on his stomach. His head was centered, and his limbs and feet were very relaxed. He was involved in a deep feeling state. He wanted contact and enjoyed when his partner gently put her hands on his hands and stroked his head.

Another person lay down with her hands on her hips and her elbows extended far out to the sides. She also had tension in her jaw and chin. When her partner tried to slightly move one of her elbows and one of her hands, the woman resisted and this developed into a fighting/struggle process. The woman's partner also touched her chin and discovered the same tension and process there.

A man lay down and immediately put something over his eyes. What could this signify? He wanted to go inside and shut out the outside world. How could you amplify this? Encourage him to go deep inside, to forget the world and go far away. Tell him that you will be with him wherever he goes but that he does not have to relate to you or the "outside" world at all.

Another person lay down with his arms slightly out to the sides; his hands were rotated slightly upward and were gently open. His head was almost imperceptibly tilted backward. This was the beginning of "going up"—a flying process!

A woman lay down, and there was a distinct tension that could be seen in the way that her feet were not relaxed but slightly bent upward. When her partner pressed against the balls of her feet, she pressed back strongly and found herself pushing something away.

3. **Get feedback.** Ask the person in the "coma" to give you feedback about the effectiveness of your amplification and bodywork abilities. The "comatose" person should answer the following:

❖ What was your inner experience?

❖ Did the hands-on interventions help to deepen or diminish the postural body experience?

❖ What would have been more helpful?

Basic Postural Awareness

Quick Review

1. Assume any posture.
2. Experiment with amplification.
3. Get feedback.

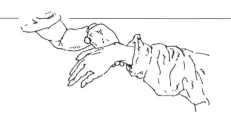

Exercise 2

Postural Awareness II

Continue your learning about postural awareness by trying the following.

Instructions (*in pairs; 15 to 20 minutes*)

1. **Try postures described in Chapter 4.** Turn to Chapter 4, Exercise 4, step 2. Together with your partner, try assuming these postures and positions of the body.

2. **Experiment with amplifying these postures.** One partner should try to amplify these various postures that her partner makes. Then switch, and the other person should try amplification.

3. **Discuss.** Discuss your learning with your partner.

Postural Awareness II

Quick Review

1. Try postures described in Chapter 4.
2. Experiment with amplifying these postures.
3. Discuss.

Exercise 3

Moving the Body and Testing the Limbs

The following exercise acquaints you with movement techniques and sensitizes your hands to muscular feedback. You test various body parts and notice subtle or more obvious movement feedback. This simple movement intervention can put you in contact with a comatose person's inner process and help him become aware of his movement potential.

Instructions *(5 minutes in the whole group; 20 minutes per person in pairs)*

1. **Demonstrate tension and relaxation.** In the middle of the whole group, one person should lie on the floor and another person should slowly raise one of his arms. The person lying down should demonstrate first a tense, stiff arm (Figure 54). Now begin again, this time demonstrating a flaccid arm as the helper raises the arm slightly (Figure 55).

2. **Do Exercise 1 in Chapter 5.** Read through the following notes, and then try the exercise in pairs.

❖ **Discovering the process in the body.** In this exercise you lift parts of the body very slowly to discover experiences in those body parts. The person's muscles are organized by an inner process the person may not yet be aware of. The touch of your hands helps bring awareness to, and facilitates the expression of, what may lie in the depths of the comatose person. It is like discovering the hidden dance inside the body that has not yet been explicitly expressed.

Even if the muscles give only a slight hint of the direction of the movement, the comatose person's inner body experience can direct you in what needs to happen. For example, imagine that you pick up the person's arm and feel a slight tendency of the arm to move outward. Use your own hands to support and encourage this motion by lightly supporting the arm underneath the wrist and elbow and gently moving your

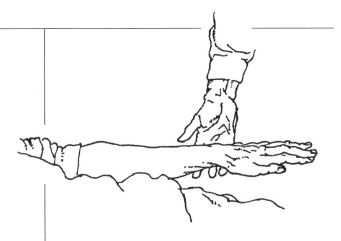

Fig. 54
A stiff arm

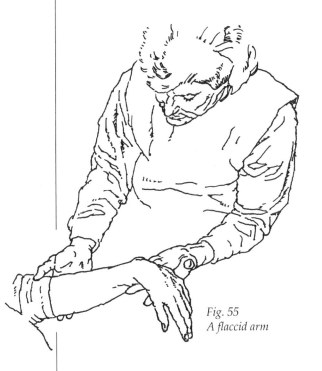

Fig. 55
A flaccid arm

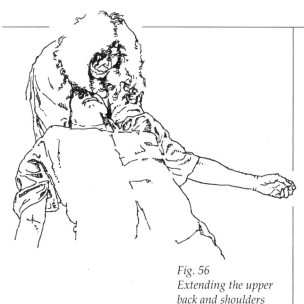

Fig. 56
Extending the upper back and shoulders

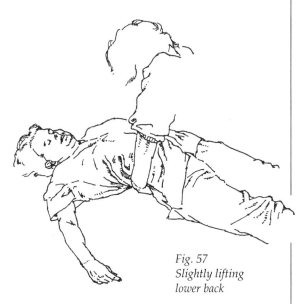

Fig. 57
Slightly lifting lower back

hands in conjunction with this outward motion. The person's inner process and movements become your guide as to the direction and quality of your movement work.

Such very slow movement allows the client to become aware of his own movement potential. He can then "direct" you with his muscles without having to have the strength to move the entire limb alone. The important thing is not your motion, but the client's direction.

These techniques are also important to try if you notice a hand, arm, leg, or head begin to move by itself. Make sure that you touch and hold the bony parts of the body because the muscles are then free to express themselves.

❖ **Additional techniques.** If there is movement in the shoulders or upper chest, you can place your hands underneath the upper back and gently extend your hands outward and lengthen the back—as long as there is no injury in this area, no difficulty with breathing and no tracheotomy—and notice any feedback to this (Figure 56).

If *breathing* is a prominent signal, you can place your hands underneath the lower back—again, making sure the back isn't injured, the breathing is unobstructed, and there is no tracheotomy—and gently press on the inhale and release on the exhale, noticing feedback (Figure 57). You can also test the *legs* by lifting and gently extending them and noticing feedback (Figure 58).

❖ **Open touch: sensitivity and feedback.** The way you touch is very important. Use an "open" touch. Your hands are saying to the comatose person, "Use my touch to sense deep processes trying to happen in your body." Use your hands to notice subtle responses in the tissues and muscles when you slightly move the person's arms, legs, head, or hand. In essence, you are using your hands sentiently to notice sometimes obvious and frequently nearly imperceptible responses and tendencies in the muscles.

In *Body Stories: A Guide to Experiential Anatomy*, Andrea Olsen describes this sense of touch as follows:

> …touch is a dialogue…. Bring your attention to the area and receive information through your hand, like a sensitive micro-

phone. You are creating a dialogue between your hand and the area being touched. In this "empty" time of not doing, you are actually bringing awareness and initiating the dialogue...[1]

As you lift a part of the body, millimeter by millimeter, notice subtle or larger feedback in the person's muscles, such as movement in a particular direction, holding, tension, weightiness, small twitches, flaccidity, shaking, or spontaneous motions. Encourage these verbally, such as by saying:

"Yes, I felt that jitter, woah! Jittering!"

If you are unsure of what you are sensing, you can say:

"Oh, I felt a little something, go ahead by yourself."

You are giving the person room to move and encouraging her to be aware and follow her experiences.

Encourage the movement through responses from your hands. For example, if you lift the arm and it begins to twitch slightly, respond by lightly jiggling your hands in response. If the arm moves slightly to the side, follow this motion with the support of your fingers underneath the elbow and wrist.

❖ **Amplification.** Amplification methods help us deepen and unfold inner experiences. Here we amplify impulses in the muscles. A helpful method for amplifying movement signals is to go with, or to slightly inhibit, the movement that is happening. (For more on movement amplification, see Chapter 11, Exercises 3 and 4.)

There are two typical responses that you can only feel with your fingers when lifting the arm, leg, or hand. Sometimes you may notice tension and lots of energy; the person is in the midst of a very wakeful, energetic state. Help the person complete this process by using your hands to go with the direction of the tension or slightly resist it. At other times, or on other days, the limb might be heavy and limp. This is most indicative of a relaxed state—of being "on vacation" and letting go. Use soothing, relaxing motions with your hands. Help the person complete this process by encouraging him to relax and enjoy letting go.

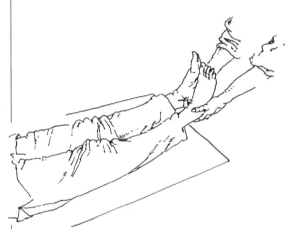

Fig. 58
Lifting and extending the legs

Note about massage and tension: In general, massage can be soothing, especially when the comatose person is in a relaxed state. Normally, when we do massage, either with a comatose person or with someone in an ordinary state of consciousness, we tell the person to let go and relax. But if there is tension in the body, you have to wonder where it goes. You can let go of tension, but it is an experience that is trying to express itself. We prefer to see tension at the surface where it is still tractable and can be worked with. The most thorough form of massage is one that allows whatever is happening in the body to express itself, whether that be relaxation or intensity. After such interactions the tension generally dissipates and the person is more relaxed than before.

*Moving the Body and
Testing the Limbs*

Quick Review

1. Demonstrate tension and relaxation.
2. Do Exercise 1 in Chapter 5.
3. Discuss.

Remember that the kinds of responses you receive may change from day to day or even during one session. Most important is your ability to adapt to the flow of what is happening. Also remember that when you are working with a comatose person, doing less is better than doing more. Follow positive feedback, try a different method if you receive no feedback, or take a break.

3. **Discuss.** Discuss your learnings with your partner.

Exercise 4

Detailed Coma Exercise

This exercise is a synthesis of all the skills you have learned to this point. You can return over and over again to this exercise for basic coma training practice. This is a long exercise, and I suggest that you take a full half-hour per person for the coma work, then fifteen minutes for discussion. After this, switch roles. The other person should lie down, and the second person should become the helper.

At the end of this exercise I include a transcript of a demonstration from a coma training seminar, which will help convey a greater sense of the flow of the work, including verbal methods and metaskills that support the techniques.

Read and discuss the following tips before beginning the exercise.

❖ **Make a time limit**. In this exercise, a time limit is especially important. It provides a framework for going into and coming out of the altered state. As the helper, let the person you are working with know when five or ten minutes remain in an exercise. Tell your partner to enjoy and follow her trance state, and that in five or ten minutes she should come out and be able to discuss her experiences with you. Make sure to save enough time for this important discussion.

❖ **Go only as far as you want to go.** For the person lying down, this exercise may bring up material that may not be close to consciousness. When you are in this role, go only as far as you want to go. Process the information with your partner in any way you feel is helpful.

❖ **Give constructive feedback.** Once again, the person who lies on the floor and imagines going into a deep trance should enjoy the process but remain awake enough to give constructive feedback to the helper—possibly during but especially after the exercise.

❖ **Experiment with becoming more free.** As you begin to make connection with someone in a coma, and after some time of being together, you no longer need to say everything you will do before you do it. You can feel a bit freer in your work.

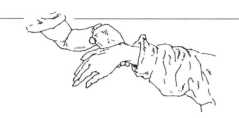

Instructions *(in pairs; 45 minutes per person: 30 minutes for the coma work, 15 minutes for discussion and note taking)*

1. **Tune in.** One person lies down and imagines she is in a coma or deep trance state. The helper should take time to tune in to the "comatose" person's state. Try to feel sentiently into the person's altered state. Notice the person's posture, any other body signals, and rate of breathing. Align yourself with this breathing rate.

2. **Get close, pace breathing, and press the wrist.** Sit near the person and again notice her rate of breathing. Adjust your breath and speech to this rhythm. Put your head close to hers, and speak just near her ear. Mumble sounds or make gentle inhaling and exhaling breaths that match the person's breathing rate. Say you are there, that you will be there for some time, and that in a moment you will touch her wrist. Press the wrist on the inhalation, release on the exhalation.

3. **Talk about following inner experience.** Put your head close to the person's ear and, speaking in the rhythm of her breath, say something like:

   "All you have to do is follow what is happening inside of you. Experiment with trusting in it, whatever it is that you might be experiencing. This will show us the way."

4. **Mention sensory channels, and respond to feedback.** Speaking in the rhythm of her breath, tell the person:

   *"You might be **feeling** things,**… you might be **seeing** things,*… or **hearing** things,*… or maybe you are **making movements**.*… If you are **feeling** something,*… then **feel** it *… if you are **seeing** something, then **look** at it *… if you are **hearing** something, then **listen** *… if you are **moving**, then follow these **movements** *…."*

   Pause a bit after mentioning each channel, and watch for feedback. Notice when you get the strongest response, and encourage the person to follow her experiences.

   For example, if you receive an especially strong response to any one sensory channel, say more about it, such as:

"Oh, seeing, yes, looking, just watch," or *"Hmmm, hearing, listening, listen closely ..."*

Recall your learnings about typical signals associated with specific channels (see Chapter 8, Exercise 6), and recommend that the person follow these experiences.

If you are unsure about channels, just encourage the person in a general way to follow what she is seeing, hearing, or feeling, or small movements that arise.

5. **Try other methods you have learned.** Try other methods you have learned until this point, watching for the moment when you gain the greatest response. Remember:

❖ To respond verbally to all signals with words or affirmative blank-access statements.

❖ To add sounds in order to create a communication system.

❖ To use your hands to test body parts and discover processes that may be taking place in the muscles.

❖ To notice and amplify postural, movement, and facial signals.

Make sure your interventions mirror the person's signals in quality and tempo.

There are many ways to amplify signals. One method is to mirror the response in different parts of the body. In this way the person can experience her process more fully. For example, if the person squeezes your hand, squeeze back in response, then gently squeeze the shoulder, the head, or the arm. If there is a tapping motion of the hand, gently tap on different parts of the body, like the elbow, knee, or shoulder. If the arm is flaccid and relaxed, perform massage-like movements and make soothing sounds as you encourage the person to relax and go on vacation.

6. **Continue to help the process unfold.** Use all the skills you have learned to help your partner unfold her experience. Be as fluid as possible and continue to focus on the verbal, touch, or movement interactions that receive the strongest feedback. Once you have really

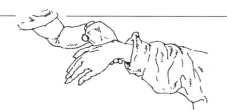

established a connection to the person's inner experience, you will feel that you are on track and that the process is flowing on its own. (See Chapter 11, Exercise 3, for more on unfolding.)

Do not get stuck with one method that isn't working. Try others. Remember, when you are actually working with a comatose person and do not gain much response, try a new method or take a break. The person may need a rest.

Remember that your sensitivity and compassion are your greatest tools.

Be sure to tell your partner in trance when she has five or ten minutes left for her inner experiences.

7. **Discuss.** After a half-hour, sit together and talk about:

❖ The "comatose" person's experiences.

❖ How these experiences might be useful to her in her everyday life.

❖ What the helper did that was useful.

❖ What could have been more helpful.

❖ The helper's experiences doing coma work.

8. **Take notes.** You and your partner should make notes about learning and experiences in your personal logs.

Detailed Coma Exercise

Quick Review

1. Tune in.
2. Get close, pace breathing, and press the wrist.
3. Talk about following inner experience.
4. Mention sensory channels, and respond to feedback.
5. Try other methods you have learned.
6. Continue to help the process unfold.
7. Discuss.
8. Take notes.

Verbatim Transcript of Detailed Coma Exercise

The following is a brief verbatim transcript of a training seminar in which the previous exercise is demonstrated with a seminar participant. I include it here because it may give you some hints regarding the flow and integration of many of the coma work methods we have learned so far. In this case, Arny is working with a man who has been in a coma two times in his life. Notice the words Arny uses, the blank-access statements, the breath work, the method of testing the head, and the special feeling behind the work.

Most important, I include this transcript to give you a sense of how to elaborate verbally about signals. I do not know how to teach this skill, other than to illustrate it here. Notice how Arny comments on the man's smile, his imaginations and feelings. I have outlined these phrases in bold print.

The student said that he had been in comas twice in his life a number of years ago. One coma resulted from mumps and meningitis and the other from pancreatitis.

Arny: Just lie down and act as if you are going into a coma. [The man lies down. Arny sits next to him on his right side, near his head, and speaks in rhythm with the man's breathing.] That's right... breathe as you're breathing... Right... Uh-huh.

I'm Arny, that's me here by your side. In a moment I will gently touch your wrist in rhythm with your breathing and then touch your elbow. Believe in the experiences in there. [Arny holds the man's wrist and follows his breathing.]

Now, while in that state, all you need to do is follow what's happening inside, trusting the experiences that you're having, whatever they might be.

You might be feeling things, or sometimes people see things, you might be hearing things, or sometimes tiny little movements happen [continuing to speak in the rate of the man's breathing and making breathing sounds now and then to this rhythm].

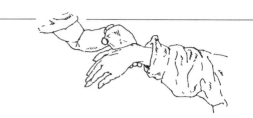

So, if you are feeling [the man takes a big breath]… yes, feeling! Or if you are seeing or hearing or moving, go right ahead and just follow these. That's right, you're doing really well. [The man swallows.] I saw that. Thoughts come your way! Just follow them. You might even experiment with believing in them… believing in the feelings and thoughts that you are having and following them.

[Arny comments to the group that people like to have input from the outside when they are deeply inside.] **Feelings and thoughts, right.** [The man swallows.] **Hmm, a little thought.** We'll just be with you while you are following things and to the best of our ability we'll help you to complete those experiences.

[The man smiles slightly.] Uh-huh… hmmm. [The man's stomach quivers a bit. Arny bends down close to him, putting his hand on the man's stomach, gently pressing as the man exhales and releasing on the inhale. The man smiles again.] **Smile, yes, it's a beautiful smile, I understand. Lovely. Smile to yourself.**

Right. Just follow experiences that are happening there. **Follow all things, even the smile.** [The man smiles again.] **Yes, that one! Sometimes people smile, sometimes grin, sometimes thoughts that go with it are important. Sometimes smiles are about certain things, sometimes just pleasures.**

[The man's lips begin to move slightly.] I see your lips began to move. There you go. [Arny now strokes the top of the man's head, then moves around to the top of the man's head and tests it by gently lifting it underneath the bottom of the skull and noticing if there is any response. The man's head and chin begin to tilt upward.] **Sometimes moving the head like this… is connected to imagination! So go ahead and follow, even if you don't know where it is going, with my hand under there.** [The man's head turns slightly to the side.] Great!

The man then makes a big smile, tilts his head up even further, and reaches up and pulls Arny toward him. Arny strokes the man's head now as they embrace.

After a few minutes, the man begins to talk about how comforted he felt and how he needs this feeling of comfort and support in his life as a whole.

The man says that, most important, he himself is a very warm and comforting person who wants to be this way toward other people. He says he has always felt this way but has been shy to express it; yet it is a deep, guiding force in his life. Arny and the man then take time to talk further about the man's coma experiences and about integrating this deep part of himself into everyday life.

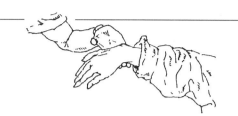

Exercise 5

Establishing Binary Communication

When someone is in a coma, it is possible to ask him questions about his needs—his inner experiences, his desires concerning medical care, about levels of pain, about life and death, and so on— if you establish a binary system of communication. *Binary* means that the comatose person can answer your questions with either a "yes" or a "no" response.

Instructions (*in pairs; 20 minutes per person*)

1. **Read preparatory notes.** Before doing the exercise, consider these notes.

   To establish communication, you first need to identify a signal that the person uses which repeats. The person may raise an eyebrow a number of times, change skin colorations frequently, take a big breath repeatedly, or occasionally squeeze your hand. Use your observational skills to notice one recurring signal.

   Following is a short description of identifying a repetitive signal while I was working with a woman in a coma.

   In the beginning of the work, the only distinguishable signal the woman was making was a faint sound, which she made a number of times. I noticed this sound and attempted to interact with it.

   > Woman: *Whhohh.*
   >
   > Amy: *Yes, "whoohh." I hear that.* [The woman makes the sound again and I continue.] *If you can hear me, make a sound.* [She takes a big breath and makes a sound again on the exhale.] *Yes, I hear that. Know I hear you... Yes. If you are there, try to make a sound, make an amazing sound, maybe only one you can hear.*
   >
   > Woman: *Mmmmm, mmm.*
   >
   > Amy: *I hear you, it's beautiful to hear you.*
   >
   > Woman: *Whoa!!*
   >
   > Amy: *Yes, yes, I hear you, I'm going to...*

Woman: *Mmmmmm ...*

Amy: *More sounds. What a beautiful voice you have!*

You can continue to develop binary communication by letting the person know that she can use that signal to communicate with you. You can increase the person's awareness of that particular signal by gently touching just in the place where the signal seems to originate. For example, touch the mouth or throat when the person is making sounds, the muscles of the eyelids when the movement of the eyelids is the determining signal, or the muscles just above the eyebrow when the eyebrow is moving. Say something like:

"Yes, you can make those sounds [or movements]. You can make those sounds [or movements] to communicate with me."

Ask whether the person can make the sound or movement again. If so, you have established a method of communication.

It is important to know that the questions you ask should be related to the person's altered state of consciousness, such as:

"Are you in pain?"

"Is it a good experience in there?"

Questions related to ordinary reality such as *"Do you remember Uncle Bill?"* are less useful. Also, questions should be closed-ended ones that can be answered with a "yes" or "no." Don't ask open-ended questions (such as *"How are you feeling?"* or *"What is happening with you?"*).

2. **Try exercise.** Turn to Chapter 5, Exercise 3, and try it with a partner.

3. **Discuss.** After ten minutes, stop and discuss the following questions together:

❖ How did you, as the helper, feel establishing binary communication?

❖ How did your partner experience your communication?

❖ According to your partner, which questions were helpful? What other questions would have been more helpful?

4. **Take notes.** Write down observations about your learning.

Establishing Binary Communication

Quick Review

1. **Read preparatory notes.**
2. **Try exercise.**
3. **Discuss.**
4. **Take notes.**

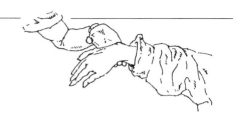

Summary of Learning from Chapter 9

❖ Be aware of the person's posture and body position, and gently amplify it through the use of touch.

❖ Use your hands to sensitively test body parts (arms, legs, head, and chin) in order to discover deep processes located in the muscles.

❖ Amplify impulses in the muscles by going with or slightly inhibiting the movement that is happening.

❖ Get feedback from your partner about the coma skills you have learned until this point.

❖ Develop binary communication by identifying a recurring signal the person can use to answer yes-or-no questions.

Note

1. Olsen, 79.

Chapter 10

W hen someone is in a coma, she is communicating in the most fundamental ways that use sounds, movement, visions, and touch. Even before these overt expressions lie deep, sentient tendencies that form the foundation from which experiences arise. All the work we do with coma relies on our ability to relate to these two basic levels of experience. The comatose person feels most understood and related to if we enter these streams of communication.

Frequently, however, edges arise when we begin to communicate in these new ways. Many people are shy about using sounds, getting close to the comatose person, working with movement, and using touch as a way of communicating. Many of us are either shy or do not know about our own sentient experiences.

Because of these edges, there is frequently a huge discrepancy between the coma helper and the client. The helper looks uptight, awkward, and limited in his access to different modes of communication. The comatose person seems to have all the options, while the helper has few!

For example, one time a helper showed a videotape of her work with a comatose woman. The woman was moving around a lot, waving her hands in the air and lifting herself up slightly from the bed. The therapist stood somewhat far away, looked a bit frozen, and responded verbally to the woman's movements but in a low tone. We encouraged the therapist, next time she would be with the comatose person, to sense the comatose person's world, to move in closer, and to use sounds that mirrored the

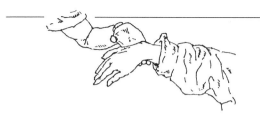

quality of the woman's motions and touch. The therapist said she was quite shy and needed to work first on her fears and edges.

The following exercises are arranged toward investigating our edges in these areas. They are geared toward an ever increasing comfort and fluidity with and a deepening of all your coma work skills and metaskills. These exercises can be informative and also fun!

Exercise 1

Sentient Inner Work with Movement and Poetry

In this exercise, we explore our openness to our own sentient experiences by focusing on movement tendencies that occur even before motion manifests overtly.[1] We will come in contact with these subtle movement impulses and help them unfold through various sensory channels with the assistance of mythic and poetic language.

One of the most effective ways of expressing sentient experiences is to speak poetically or mythically about them. It is important to practice creating poetic language because many people in comatose states are experiencing deep mythic processes and seem to relate to the use of poetry, mythic images, and song, which embellish and further inner experiences. Yet, many of us have edges in using mythic or poetic verse.

Many of us are very shy to speak poetically or to sing songs. We become blocked, feel awkward or uncomfortable. Why? Responses from my classes include the following:

❖ *I'm shy to express myself in this way because I feel too vulnerable.*

❖ *I just feel silly.*

❖ *This is expressing something on a soul level. I'm shy to share that.*

❖ *I'm not supported to be like this in everyday life.*

❖ *People try to keep me away from this poetic part of myself.*

❖ *It is too intimate, and it scares me.*

- ❖ *I don't feel met in this mythical place in myself and therefore I don't share it with others. It seems too feeling or romantic.*
- ❖ *It's too deep to really believe in.*

Here you will have the opportunity to explore edges about your sentient experiences and the creation of poetry and song.

Instructions (*each person alone; guided by someone in the group; 15 minutes for the exercise, 15 minutes for discussion with partner*)

1. **Sit in a comfortable position.** Find a comfortable spot and go inside yourself. Simply be with yourself. Relax. Your eyes can be open, but it is better if they are closed.

2. **Be unknowing.** Assume a special attitude of "unknowingness." That is, try to assume an empty and open mind, one that feels unfocused and unknowing. This may give you a special relaxed, drifting feeling in your head in which you do not have to focus on anything. Your focus is diffuse and open.

3. **Notice a movement tendency.** Now, notice any slight tendency in your body to move, even before the movement happens, even before it is expressed overtly. Sense this tendency. Get in contact with it. Believe in it. Open up to it as a mystery trying to unfold, even without knowing what it is. Notice whether you have edges to following this "unknown" experience.

4. **Unfold.** Feel this movement tendency. Now let it begin to express itself in movement. Give it time and space to show itself. Now make a picture which mirrors or represents that movement experience. Look at that picture. Stay with the image, feeling, and movement, and allow these to unfold in their own creative way.

5. **Add words, poetry, or song.** Now, try to translate that overall experience into words or poetry. Use mythic or poetic words to describe and express this experience to yourself. Free yourself to wax poetic! Or hum a tune or make up a song that gives musical voice to this experience.

For example, one woman experienced the wind blowing through her bones and suddenly imagined that her bones disintegrated. She then felt there was nothing at all except a profound silence. She created the following poem: "A hawk flies as the moon shines on the sand... then there was nothing."

If you experience a deep relaxed state, you might say something like "Going far, far away, deep down and away ... Drift, drift, to the sea...." Or create and sing a song about floating away on a gentle breeze.

6. **Notice whether the experience wants to transform ordinary life**. Now simply notice if the experience you just had would like to transform your ordinary life in some way, or if it wants to simply be experienced.

7. **Discuss your experience with a partner**.

❖ Share your experience.

❖ Does this experience want to influence you in any way in your ordinary life, or does it want to stay in that sentient world and simply be experienced?

❖ What mythic words or song did you use to describe your experience? Was this hard to do? Were you shy? What would help you feel less shy?

❖ Did you feel shy, at any time, to go deeper into your altered state? Was it hard to be unknowing and follow what was happening with an open, beginner's mind?

❖ Generally, how open do you feel to your own altered states? What would help you open up more to your inner sentient experiences?

Note: We have found that, sometimes when you work with a comatose person, his sentient experience is trying to regenerate everyday life. You sense that he is reaching toward ordinary reality and would like to bridge these two worlds. At other times, the person needs time in this altered state and would like support in following inner experiences without having to relate to ordinary life. Many people in coma may be searching for this chance to go deeply inside without having to relate to ordinary reality. This step helps ponder these two realms of experience. (See Chapter 12 for more on this topic.)

Sentient Inner Work with Movement and Poetry

Quick Review

1. **Sit in a comfortable position.**
2. **Be unknowing.**
3. **Notice a movement tendency.**
4. **Unfold.**
5. **Add words, poetry, or song.**
6. **Notice whether the experience wants to transform ordinary life.**
7. **Discuss your experience with a partner.**

Exercise 2

Investigating Shyness and Making Sounds

You may have been surprised when you tried making sounds while doing the exercises in Chapter 9. Many people find it very difficult and "edgy" to make nonsensical sounds, especially when communicating with someone who is not "talking" in the accustomed way. Shyness and inhibition about making sounds surface in about eighty percent of my students. For many of us, making sounds is like breaking a cultural communication taboo. We feel we should act like adults, speak intelligently, and not make strange noises!

How can we find the inner freedom necessary for communicating with people in coma? Do you remember using all sorts of sounds to communicate with, soothe, and play with a child? These modes of communicating are not only important for interacting with children, but are the very basis of sensitive communication.

Use this exercise to experiment. Although it may seem silly at first, the exercise will help you gain access to and ease with communication methods that are central to your coma work. Paradoxically, class participants often enjoy this exercise the most!

Instructions *(in pairs; 10 minutes per person)*

1. **One person acts like a child.** One of you should start to act like a baby or very young child.

2. **Experiment with using sounds.** The helper should experiment with communicating in a way that she would with a "real" child. Notice that the helper must communicate in nonsensical sounds, tones, song, movements, and touch.

3. **Communicate with more sound.** If the "child" also makes sounds, the helper should try to amplify those sounds by repeating them and adding on other sounds.

4. **Notice the strongest feedback.** The helper notices where the most energy is, that is, when or where the "child" responds with the strongest signal—in touch, sound, or movement. The helper should stay

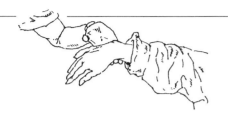

focused on this element, amplify it, and deepen it through creative communication. There is no right way. Experiment. Have fun!

5. **Investigate shyness.** If you feel shy and unable to communicate in this way, switch modes. Your partner should come out of her childlike state and help you find out what stops you from making sounds, as follows:

❖ Let an image form of "who" within you inhibits you.

❖ Explore the conflict between yourself and this inner figure. For example, a woman had a conflict with a part of herself that said she would look ridiculous if she made sounds. This figure said she should act like a mature adult. The woman responded to her inner figure by saying that it was not ridiculous to make sounds if they would be helpful to another person and that, furthermore, it would feel great to be free enough to make these noises and movements and to be so spontaneous. She hated feeling so restricted and uptight! Together with her partner, the woman continued this dialogue until a resolution emerged which both parts could agree on. She was allowed to be spontaneous half of the day but then had to be very studious and adult-like the rest of the time!

6. **Discuss and take notes.** Afterwards, discuss the exercise with your partner and write down your experiences in your personal log in the back of the book.

❖ How did you feel making sounds? Were you shy?

❖ How free do you feel in this kind of communication?

❖ If you felt inhibited, what inhibited you? How did you resolve this conflict?

❖ What was it like to be a child or a baby?

Investigating Shyness and Making Sounds

Quick Review

1. One person acts like a child.
2. Experiment with using sounds.
3. Communicate with more sound.
4. Notice the strongest feedback.
5. Investigate shyness.
6. Discuss and take notes.

Exercise 3

Exploring Edges of Intimacy and Contact

Coma work methods depend on your ability to be close to, and in physical contact with, the comatose person. However, many helpers have edges or inhibitions about intimacy and contact, particularly when interacting with someone in a deep, altered state of consciousness. Many of us are timid and afraid to put our cheek near the other's cheek, to talk intimately, and to communicate with touch.

You may ask, "Is it appropriate to get so close to the comatose person and even touch her in respectful ways when I don't even know the person?" We have never met any comatose person who did not respond well to intimate contact when the helper introduced herself first and held good intentions. Comatose people appreciate it when someone sensitively communicates and helps follow their inner processes.

A thought to consider: comas can be lonely places, both emotionally and physically. One hospice consultant commented to me that, in her experience, people in coma need a lot of body contact and tactile stimulation, especially if they have been in the hospital for long periods.[2] Many of these people are frequently alone and have had very little tactile contact, other than the touch associated with medical care. A loving touch, a warm hand or cheek, can bring warmth and friendship into this isolated spot.

Remember that the experiences people go through in comas are similar to our own, but more intense. Yet, all of us go through deep experiences at one time or another in our lives. This knowledge gives you the sense that everyone, in a way, is part of your family and is really not that different from you.

One of the best ways to work with shyness is *not* to ignore it; instead, respect it and explore it in greater detail. In this exercise, take the time to explore your edges about touch and intimacy. Don't jump over your inhibitions. Use this exercise to find out more about yourself.

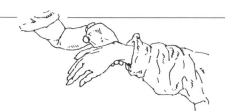

Instructions *(in pairs; 15 minutes per person)*

1. **Slowly move closer.** One person lies down. When your partner takes the coma role, you as the helper should sit near her. Slowly begin to move even nearer to her. Move so that your face and your cheek come closer and closer to the ear of the person on the floor.

2. **Notice your feelings.** As you get closer to the "comatose" person, use your awareness to notice all the subtle fluctuations in your feelings. Notice even the slightest twinges of discomfort, shyness, fear, and so on.

3. **Talk about the experience, and identify beliefs.** Your partner should now sit up and discuss with you your feelings in response to the intimacy and contact. Are your edges due to:

❖ Shyness about being with someone in an altered state?

❖ Shyness about contact in general?

❖ Shyness around intimacy?

Try to identify a belief system that inhibits your freedom in this (these) area(s). For example, "You shouldn't be so close to someone, it's wrong," "Being so intimate is only for lovers," or "You should stay away from someone in such a weird state that you can't understand."

4. **Imagine what would make you more comfortable.** Imagine what might make you more comfortable, such as more comfort with your own altered states, working on your abuse issues, spending time becoming more comfortable with movement and touch, or gaining more practice.

If you did not find any edges, congratulations! Explore what it is about you that makes you so comfortable. How did you learn this? Have you always been that way? Why?

5. **Try again.** Now your partner should lie down once again. As the helper, again approach the person, getting close and then closer, noticing whether anything has changed in your feelings.

6. **Discuss.** Talk about your experiences with your partner.

Exploring Edges of Intimacy and Contact

Quick Review

1. Slowly move closer.
2. Notice your feelings.
3. Talk about the experience, and identify beliefs.
4. Imagine what would make you more comfortable.
5. Try again.
6. Discuss.

Exercise 4

Developing Loving Touch

The kind of touch you use in coma work is very important. The best touch is a loving touch in which your hands sense the slightest responses in the person's muscles, tissues, and skin. Your hands seem to perceive sentient processes even before they emerge. You notice the energy between the two of you and feel deeply connected to the other person in a nonverbal way.

When you touch the person, your hands should convey an openness, which the person can use as a means of contact. This openness can help the person express her body process. This is like a blank access with touch!

How do you learn this sense of touch? Practice helps. There are also many bodywork and massage techniques that teach you how to develop sensitivity with your hands when touching someone else.[3]

In this exercise, experiment with touching your partner in a loving, responsive way. This is a purely feeling-oriented exercise, so take the time to experiment with it, focusing solely on the quality of your touch rather than your skills.

Instructions (*in pairs; 5 minutes per person*)

1. **Sit with a partner.** Sit next to your partner.

2. **Touch your partner.** Use your hands to touch your partner on the shoulder or the hand.

3. **Experiment with a loving touch.** Now focus your attention on the quality of your touch. Experiment with generating a loving touch, in which you sense the energy flow between the two of you. Your hands should convey an openness your partner can use to express herself. Try to feel the nonverbal "energetic" link with your partner.

4. **Notice any feedback.** With your hands, notice any physical feedback from your partner's muscles, tissues, or skin. There may be almost imperceptible reactions, quivers, larger movements, warmth, gentle

movements toward or away from your hands. Be sensitive to even the most minimal responses.

5. **Discuss.** Discuss your experience of touching and your partner's experience of receiving that contact.

Exercise 5

Egyptian Bodywork

The following bodywork exercise gives you a glimpse of how the person in coma is in the midst of dreams, fantasies, mythic experiences, or a combination of these. It is excerpted from a seminar Arny and I gave on the Tibetan and Egyptian *Books of the Dead*. These *Books of the Dead* offer methods for accompanying individuals while they are dying and even after death.

The ancient Egyptians used special methods in which they worshipped parts of the body as if they were inhabited by goddesses and gods in need of appreciation and respect. This exercise involves developing a worshipful feeling for the body. It helps cultivate the metaskill of caring for and appreciating each individual's unique body process and the special communication emanating from parts of the body.

Instructions *(in pairs; 20 minutes per person)*

1. **One person lies down.** One person lies down and pretends that he is in a deep trance.

2. **Massage.** As the helper, gently massage the hands, head, or feet (or a combination of these) to relax the person.

3. **Speak to the body.** Now begin talking to the different parts of the body, addressing these parts as gods and goddesses. Say something like:

   "Oh great goddess of the shoulder [or other body part], you are wondrous! Amazing what you are able to do and what you have done!"

4. **Notice any responses.** Notice whether the limbs or any areas of the body spontaneously move or respond as you speak to them. Notice deep breaths, twitches, slight movements, and so on. Encourage this part of the body, this goddess or god, to express itself. Welcome this spirit into life, as a highly respected being:

   "Oh great hand, welcome to life, express yourself as you please, you are a great goddess that we will follow."

5. **Help the process unfold as follows:**

   ❖ By encouraging or amplifying the movement that is emerging and letting the process express itself in its unique way.

   ❖ By asking your partner for visions, sounds, or fantasies that accompany the unfolding process. Perhaps the goddess will come to life and speak about herself.

6. **Discuss the experience.** Afterwards, discuss the experience with your partner as follows:

   ❖ What does this experience mean for his everyday life?

   ❖ Was this experience in any way connected to other important experiences in his past?

7. **Get feedback from your partner.** The "comatose" person should give feedback about the metaskills or feeling attitudes of the helper.

Egyptian Bodywork

Quick Review

1. One person lies down.
2. Massage.
3. Speak to the body.
4. Notice any responses.
5. Help the process unfold.
6. Discuss the experience.
7. Get feedback from your partner.

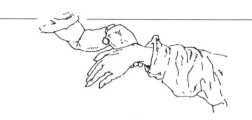

Summary of Learning from Chapter 10

❖ Comatose people express themselves through fundamental communication methods including sentient tendencies, sound, movement, vision, and touch. You will need to join these communication methods as well.

❖ Common edges of the helper include shyness about following sentient and unknown experiences, using poetry and song, making sounds, fear about getting physically close to the comatose person, and shyness about using movement and touch. Explore your edges in these areas.

❖ Practice opening up to and exploring your sentient experiences, subtle tendencies that exist before overt expression.

❖ Comatose people appreciate your intimate contact when it is made in a sensitive, loving way.

❖ The kinds of experiences comatose people are going through are not very different from our own.

❖ Explore your own edges about making sounds by practicing communicating with a child.

❖ Experiment with physical closeness. Explore any shyness you may feel about intimacy.

❖ Learn to respect the body's natural process by worshiping it like a goddess or a god.

Notes

1. Adapted from a seminar called "Lucid Dreaming" that Arny and I gave in Oregon and England in 1996 and 1997. See Arny's forthcoming books, *Mastermind* and *Twenty-four Hour Lucid Dreaming*, for more exercises and details of sentient awareness.
2. Thanks to Gerri Haynes for her insights here.
3. For example, see Aminah Raheem's *Process-Oriented Acupressure*, Fritz Smith's *Inner Bridges: Zero Balancing*, and Andrea Olsen's *Body Stories* (79, 80-81), for descriptions of various kinds of touch.

This chapter begins with general training exercises in body and movement work that provide greater ease in, and enhance your abilities with, coma work. You will become more familiar with hands-on bodywork methods and movement techniques that you can apply to your work. Exercise 5 returns to a longer coma exercise in which you can integrate coma methods learned in earlier chapters, as well as experiment with using your intuition in your work. Exercise 6 presents a method for studying a videotape of coma practice.

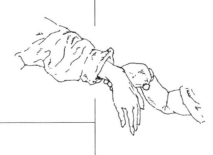

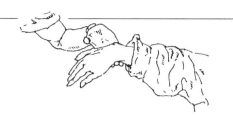

Exercise 1

Sentience in Movement

Your ability to sensitively use the body and movement techniques described in this chapter depends on your increasing ability to notice sentient tendencies before they manifest overtly. To get in contact with this awareness and as inner preparation for the next exercise, briefly repeat the inner work exercise on movement and sentience.

Instructions *(5 minutes all together)*

1. **Repeat sentient movement exercise.** Look back to Chapter 10, Exercise 1. Briefly repeat only steps 1 through 3. Unfold this experience in any way you like for a few minutes.

2. **Ask about openness**. Ask yourself how open you are to inner processes. Are you able to stay open to what is happening even if you do not completely understand it at first? Are you able to have a beginner's mind toward your experiences?

Sentience in Movement

Quick Review

1. Repeat sentient movement exercise.
2. Ask about openness.

Exercise 2

Sentient Touch and Sculpting the Face

In this exercise, use your hands as a fine sentient instrument to sense subtle processes, which may or may not be apparent on the surface. You will use a technique we call sculpting in which you use your hands like a sensitive sculptor or potter to discover, and help your partner get in touch with, processes happening in the musculature of the face. (In Chapter 12 we will explore specific methods for working with processes in the face, particularly in relationship to brain injury.)

Experiment with following the person's facial process even if you do not know where it is going, but trusting in its wisdom. Your partner may not even be aware of these experiences until you put your hands on her face.

Instructions *(in pairs; 15 minutes per person)*

1. **Sit opposite your partner, and observe.** Sit across from your partner, whose eyes are either closed or open. The helper should begin noticing her partner's face, the bone structure, facial lines, tensions, wrinkles, indentations, flaccid or taut skin, color variations, or anything else that catches her attention.

2. **Use sentient touch.** Now using your fingers and hands, begin to touch the person's face, drawing your hands along the lines, muscles, skin, or the elements that caught your attention (Figure 59). Use your hands sensitively, but not so lightly that the person cannot feel her inner facial experiences. Use a sentient touch in which you try to sense any tendencies, processes that may be occurring in the face even before they emerge.

3. **Notice feedback.** Notice feedback you receive to your touch as your hands meet and interact with the musculature of the face. Perhaps the person will tense her face more, sigh in certain moments, begin to move her jaw, or the like.

4. **Amplify.** Use your hands to amplify the experience that is emerging. Go with or slightly against the responses of the face. Think of this as

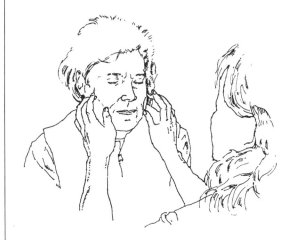

Fig. 59
Sentiently touching the face

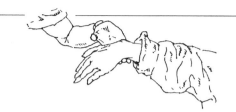

being like a dance that is developing between you. Use sounds or words to embellish the process. Creatively unfold this experience together in any way you like.

5. **Discuss.** Afterwards, discuss your own sentient touch ability and the inner experience of your partner.

For the helper:

❖ Were you, as the helper, able to sense the sentient experience in your partner's face before it expressed itself overtly?

❖ If your guess was wrong, could you let go of your ideas and simply follow the process that was trying to unfold?

For the person being touched:

❖ Talk about your inner experience.

❖ How did you experience your partner's touch? Did it help you get in contact with inner experiences in the face?

❖ Would another kind of touch have helped more?

Sentient Touch and Sculpting the Face

Quick Review

1. **Sit opposite your partner, and observe.**
2. **Use sentient touch.**
3. **Notice feedback.**
4. **Amplify.**
5. **Discuss.**

Exercise 3

Sculpting the Back

In this exercise we extend the method of sculpting, applying it to the back and the full body. This will help you combine hands-on body-work and movement techniques and gain greater ease in working with your hands. The goals in this exercise are as follows:

❖ To sense your partner's inner body process.

❖ To help your partner feel his body and muscles.

❖ To discover particular body areas and muscles that may have a particular expression or experience in them.

❖ To increase the sensitivity in those body areas so that the person can get in touch with, follow, and deepen these inner experiences.

Make sure to ask your partner first whether she has any physical limitations or difficulties, such as osteoporosis or other movement inhibitions. If so, be careful to use a gentler touch, and proceed only as far as is comfortable for your partner.

Instructions *(in pairs; 20 minutes per person)*

1. **Place hands on partner's back.** In standing position, go behind your partner and put your hands gently on her upper back (Figure 60). Your hands, in essence, convey an open or blank question that helps the person get in contact with her body process.

2. **Partner recalls and moves to dream image.** Ask your partner to call to mind an image or figure that appeared recently in one of her dreams. She should then begin to move as if she were that dream image or figure. For example, if the image is of a bear, ask her to begin to move a little bit like a bear.

3. **Sculpt.** As your partner moves, use your hands to help her feel, even more, the motions she is making. Don't be afraid to use a firm contact if your partner is in good physical condition. Imagine again that you are a sculptor who is helping her creation emerge.

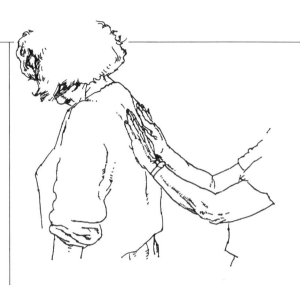
Fig. 60
Hands on the back

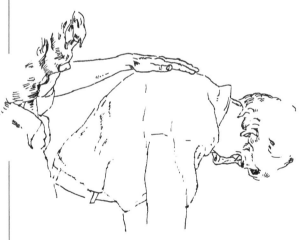
Fig. 61
Moving hands in concert with the direction of the person's movement

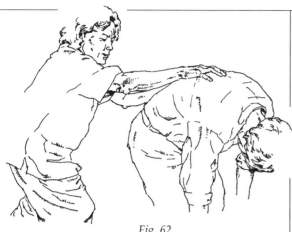

Fig. 62
*Moving hands in opposition
to the person's movement*

You can amplify your partner's movement experiences by moving your hands in concert with, and also slightly against, the direction her movement is going. Use you hands as follows:

❖ Move your hands in concert with the body motions. For example, if your partner bends forward, you can follow the movement in the direction it is going by running your hands along the back—from the lower back to the upper back—while the person leans forward (Figure 61).

❖ Move your hands in the opposite direction of the motion of the body giving just a hint of resistance. If the person is leaning forward, run your hand along the back from the upper back to the lower back giving slight resistance (Figure 62). Here, you are slightly interrupting a movement signal in order to increase its impulse.

❖ Put your hands on the lever point (the hips in this case), and use a rotating motion to give more sensation and assistance to this bending motion (Figure 63). The same principle can be applied to the lever points of the arms by touching the elbows and shoulders (Figure 64).

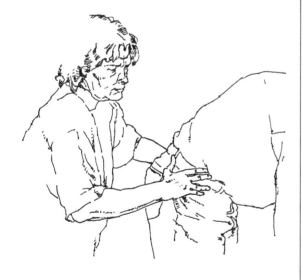

Fig. 63
*Working with the lever
point of the hips*

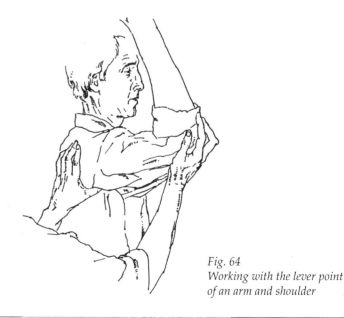

Fig. 64
*Working with the lever point
of an arm and shoulder*

❖ If the person's head begins to move, place your hands on the person's shoulders and neck. This helps the person feel her neck movements and sense which way the head would like to go. You can then gently stretch the neck muscles in the direction the head is going, or slightly go against the muscles by drawing your hand down the muscles in the opposite direction of the movement (Figure 65).

❖ If the head moves from side to side, put your hands on both sides of the head and give slight resistance.

❖ If the person takes big breaths, use your hands to sculpt the bony part of the upper chest, shoulders, and back (Figure 66).

Use your intuition and knowledge of the body and its muscular system to inform your work. It is helpful to imagine what would feel good to you if you were the mover. What would help you to gain more awareness of your body movements and to complete them? (See Figures 67-69 for more images of sculpting.)

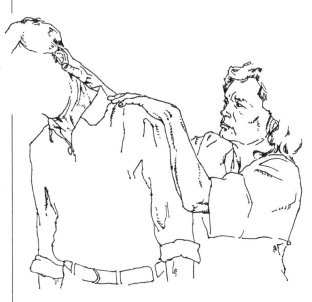

Fig. 65
Using hands on the neck to amplify head motion

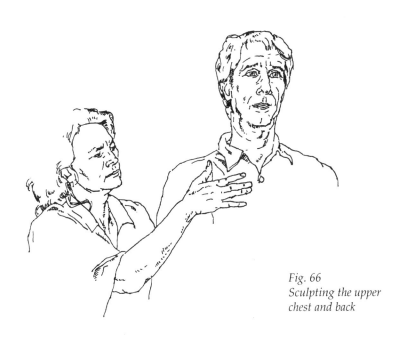

Fig. 66
Sculpting the upper chest and back

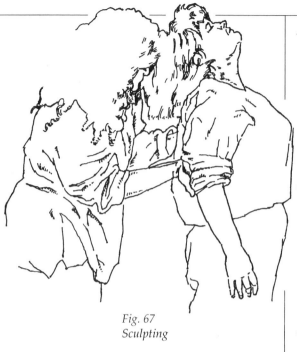

Fig. 67
Sculpting

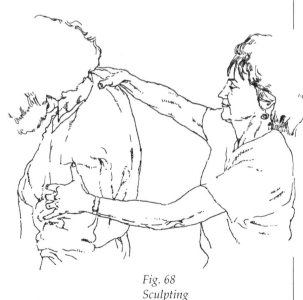

Fig. 68
Sculpting

Coma, A Healing Journey

4. **Notice new movements.** Notice whether a new movement pattern emerges, repeats, or disappears (or a combination of these occurs). Ask your partner if she would like to focus on this movement and explore it.

One of the goals of movement work is to identify secondary movement processes. That is, while the person is identifying with a particular theme in a given moment (primary movement process—in this case, the original dream image), there may also be small indications of a new process (secondary movement) trying to emerge.

❖ For example, let's say you begin to move like a bear in a slow way with hunched shoulders. This is your intention and therefore your momentary primary process. Suddenly you make a quick clawing motion with a hand, but then return again to your slow movement, only to quickly make this clawing motion again at another point. We call the unexpected clawing motion secondary. It is unintentional and surprising. A movement worker would encourage you to return to the clawing motion and help you explore and unfold it further.

❖ Here is another example. Let's say you are walking. Your intention is to walk; therefore this movement is primary. As you walk, you stumble slightly. Your helper could assist you in exploring this secondary stumbling motion further by asking you to repeat it in a safe manner, perhaps in slow motion, then allowing the movement to extend itself, to express itself even further.

Through the contact with your hands you, as the helper, may notice a new, secondary movement theme emerging in your partner. Perhaps the person suddenly begins to move against your hands; perhaps she suddenly lunges deeply or begins to tremble. When this happens, simply encourage the person, both physically and verbally, to follow these motions.

If these secondary motions suddenly disappear, or if they continually repeat themselves, the person may be at a movement edge. This means she may feel shy about completing these new motions. No matter what state of consciousness any of us is in, we all have edges. When you begin to express something new but become shy and tentative about it, you are at an edge. Work with edges by asking your partner if she would like to return to these movements, focus her attention on them, and let them unfold more fully.

Even if you do not notice a secondary movement process, the most important element here is to gain practice with using your hands through the technique of sculpting.

5. **Unfold using channel changes.** Continue sculpting until it seems that the person is on track—that she is connected to a movement story that is unfolding. Encourage your partner to continue to follow her movements and then to change channels in order to give more depth and color to the "story." Ask her to make sounds that go along with her movements or to visualize an image of what she is doing. (The original dream image may have changed.) Now, as she continues to move, suggest that she verbally tell you a story about the unfolding experience.

❖ Here is an example. A woman began to move to the image of the ocean, which she had dreamed about the night before. As her partner used his hands to sculpt the woman's back as she moved, she began to push forward slightly with her shoulders. The helper came in front of the woman and slightly resisted her shoulder motions until the woman began pushing even harder with her shoulders and then her hands. She pushed against her partner and made grunting sounds and then shouts, saying, "I want to be free! Let me out!" Then she saw an image of a little girl who was in a room that was much too small for her. As she moved, she told the story of a girl who possessed a great deal of creativity but who never had the space or support to express herself fully. The woman's partner helped her go more deeply into the various aspects of this story, including the kinds of things inhibiting her in her life, and her creativity, as well as discussing what this story could mean for her life as a whole.

6. **Discuss.** Talk together about this experience.

❖ Ask your partner what this experience might mean for her everyday life.

❖ Your partner should give you feedback about your sculpting techniques.

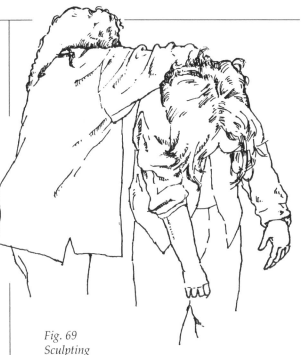

Fig. 69
Sculpting

Sculpting the Back

Quick Review

1. **Place hands on partner's back.**
2. **Partner recalls and moves to dream image.**
3. **Sculpt.**
4. **Notice new movements.**
5. **Unfold using channel changes.**
6. **Discuss.**

Exercise 4

Movement Amplification

This exercise is geared toward gaining more fluidity and comfort in working with and deepening movement processes. We will add to the movement amplification techniques we have learned until this point and begin, this time, from a reclining position. These methods can be adapted to working with comatose people.

Instructions *(in pairs; 15 minutes per person)*

1. **Partner lies down on the floor.** Ask your partner to lie on the floor.

2. **Partner begins to move.** The person on the floor should notice how he feels and begin to move according to these feelings. He may begin to make various movements, such as:

❖ Turning his head, knees, or whole body to the side.

❖ Stretching his toes forward.

❖ Lifting his arms.

❖ Tilting his head backward.

❖ Bending his knees.

❖ Arching his back.

3. **Use amplification techniques.** Use any of the following movement amplification methods to encourage, follow, and unfold the movement process:

❖ Follow the direction of the movement by going in the same direction with your hands.

❖ Go against the direction of the movement slightly with your hands. For example, if one of the legs pushes outward, use your hands to press back (Figure 70).

❖ Use your hands underneath the arms, legs, knees, elbows, or head to lightly support and follow the movement.

❖ Use sculpting techniques.

❖ When one part of the body moves, help other parts of the body do the same movement. For example, if one arm is moving up and down,

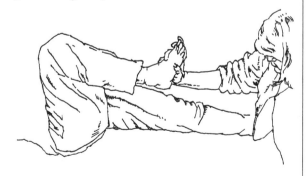

Fig. 70
Amplifying by gently pressing
against the leg as it pushes outward

move one of the person's legs or the head gently up and down as well. (See Exercise 5 below and also Chapter 12, where we will study this method in greater detail.)

❖ Encourage movements verbally with blank-access words and sounds.

❖ Add other sensory channels, such as images or sounds, to mirror the movement experience.

❖ Notice two parts to the movement. A helpful tip is that every movement is in relationship to another movement or object, even if the counterpart is only gravity. Therefore you can fill in the "invisible" part. Following are some examples.

If someone pushes out strongly with his arms, he is pushing against something else. When someone's head turns in your direction, it may be you that he is turning toward. If someone is turning over into the fetal position, the counterpart may be someone who is stroking and caring for him. If the person's mouth is puckered, it may want to touch or kiss something. If the person's head is moving back and forth from side to side, it may want resistance on both sides to feel its impulse more fully.

Try to fill in the hidden or implicit part. If a person's hand is slightly raised, facing down and gently stroking the air with its fingers, there may be something underneath that the hand is stroking. Try putting your hand underneath and see what happens. Peter (see Chapter 1) moved one of his fingers in a rhythmic motion. It turned out that this finger motion was trying to conduct a symphony. We sang along in time to his motion!

Try to guess the counterpart of a motion, express it, and notice whether this helps the movement unfold. Discover the hidden dance![1]

❖ Ask the person to tell a story about the process that is unfolding through movement.

4. **Discuss.** Explore your experience with your partner. What was helpful? What would have been more helpful?

5. **Take notes.** Jot down notes in your personal log on what you learned about movement work.

Movement Amplification

Quick Review

1. Partner lies down on the floor.
2. Partner begins to move.
3. Use amplification techniques.
4. Discuss.
5. Take notes.

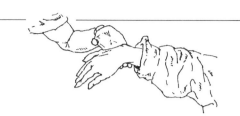

Exercise 5

Coordinated Movement: A Personal Experiment

One method of amplification is to take what is happening in one part of the body and help the person experience that process more fully by expanding it to other areas of the body. This method helps the person unfold her experience and gain a sense of congruency throughout the body.

This technique also helps the comatose person connect parts of the body that she may now have trouble connecting, particularly if brain injury has occurred. Aspects of rehabilitation rely on this technique. We will go into this more in depth in Chapter 12.

Ordinarily, we experience a sense of congruency and coordination in our movements, yet this flawless interaction is usually taken for granted. To get in touch with this innate unity, explore the following exercise, in which you discover how body parts, muscles, and movement are interconnected.[2] Once you have a thorough feeling for these connections, you will be better able to assist these connections in others.

Instructions *(alone; for 10 minutes; then discuss with a partner)*

1. **Lie down on the floor.**

2. **Experiment with movement.** For a few minutes experiment with different kinds of simple movements. For example, raise one of your arms, take a big breath, open and close your mouth, rotate one foot outward.

3. **Choose a movement.** Now choose one of those movements to study.

4. **Make inner connections.** Make the simple motion again, and use your inner sensing to feel what other body parts would naturally move in relation to this original movement. For example, let's say you choose raising an arm. Raise the arm and ask yourself internally, "Which other parts of my body feel connected to this movement?" That is, which parts of the body would also like to move in concert with this raised arm?

Try lifting the other arm at the same time. Try lifting a leg. Lift the head. Explore which additional movements *feel* right, which movements feel as if they want to express themselves together.

5. **Choose a new movement.** Now choose a different movement or experience, such as taking a deep breath. Notice which body parts would like to move naturally with this deep breath. Experiment and note the effects.

6. **Discuss.** When you are finished, share your experiences and observations with someone else in your group.

7. **Take notes.** Make notes about your personal learning regarding body connections. Sketch quick pictures to remind yourself of the body connections you discovered.

Coordinated Movement:
A Personal Experiment

Quick Review

1. **Lie down.**
2. **Experiment with movement.**
3. **Choose a movement.**
4. **Make inner connections.**
5. **Choose a new movement.**
6. **Discuss.**
7. **Make notes.**

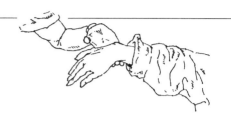

Exercise 6

Connecting Breath, Movement, and Sound: A Personal Experiment

In the following exercise you not only experience movement connections in the body, but also the connection between movement, breath, and sound. The acts of moving, breathing, and making sounds are intimately intertwined. Sound reverberates throughout the body, much as breathing accompanies the various movements that we make. To feel this connection, try the following exercise yourself.

Instructions *(alone; first standing up and then lying down; experiment for 10 minutes; discuss for 10 minutes with a partner)*

1. **Stand and make a movement.** Stand erect and make any movement you like. You might feel like making a large movement such as bending your entire torso or something so slight as moving one finger.

2. **Add breath and sound.** Do the movement again, this time accompanying it with your breath, inhaling and exhaling in a way that seems to escort the movement naturally and fluidly.

3. **Add sounds.** Now add sounds that mirror this movement and breath experience. Notice how these experiences create a growing sense of congruency or unity throughout the body.

4. **Amplify.** Intensify the experience you are having by increasing the experience to include the movement of your whole body. For example, imagine you began with the movement of your head dropping forward. You added breath and sound that mirrored this dropping movement. Now amplify this experience by dropping forward, not only with your head but also with your arms, knees, and torso, as you continue with sound and breath.

5. **Begin again with breath.** Start over this time, beginning with your breath. Take a deep breath. Discover what movements would connect to this kind of breathing— such as raising your shoulders and arms and rising to your toes as you inhale. Add sounds to your breath and movement.

6. **Begin again with sound.** Start again, this time making any kind of sound that feels right in the moment. Now add motions and breathing patterns that flow congruently with this sound. For example, if you make a strong "Ho!" sound, use your breath to amplify the intensity of the sound while making strong pushing movements with your arms and then other parts of your body.

7. **Try steps 1 through 6 lying down.**

8. **Discuss.** Share your experiences with a team worker.

Connecting Breath, Movement, and Sound: A Personal Experiment

Quick Review

1. Stand and make a movement.
2. Add breath.
3. Add sounds.
4. Amplify.
5. Begin again with breath.
6. Begin again with sound.
7. Try steps 1 through 6 lying down.
8. Discuss.

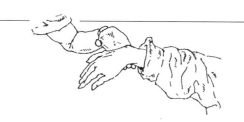

Exercise 7

Unfolding, Edges, and Intuition

The following exercise helps you integrate and review some of the coma work methods you have learned until this point. Use this exercise to focus on increasing your fluidity with the various coma work skills and metaskills.

This exercise also adds a number of new elements. You will focus on the ability to help inner processes unfold, to notice and work with edges, and to use your intuition.

Instructions (*in pairs; 25 minutes for the experiential part; 10 minutes for discussion*)

1. **Partner lies down on floor.** Your partner should lie down and imagine that he is in a deep trance state or coma. Tune in. Approach him and pace his breathing, speaking on the exhale, and suggest that he follow his inner experiences and sensory channels.

2. **Notice signals, and respond.** Watch for minimal signals, and respond to them. Use sounds and blank access statements that mirror these experiences.

3. **Test body parts, and notice responses.** Test body parts to notice whether the person is relaxed, tense, or responds to your touch. Amplify the overall body posture with the use of your hands. If you want, use binary communication by noticing and using a repetitive signal to ask the person questions.

4. **Unfold.** Follow the person's natural process by using any of the body work and movement techniques previously described. Notice moments when you get the most response, and try to help the process unfold.

Unfolding means that you are on track, that you have caught the flow of the person's process, joined his "stream," and are helping it express itself. How do you know when you are on track? This is difficult to describe for it is a matter of feeling. Here are some answers from my students, which may be of help to you:

❖ You get a response a few times and begin to communicate back and forth.

❖ There is excitement in the breathing and movement responses.

❖ You have the feeling that something lights on fire, that the process is spontaneously generating itself.

❖ You sense that you are in the middle of a story that is evolving.

❖ You sense a continual energetic stream, even if it is a quiet one.

❖ You have the intuitive sense or feeling of connection.

❖ It feels like there is a dance happening between the two of you.

❖ Attention becomes less random and more focused in the helper and in the "comatose" person.

❖ One thing easily follows the next—a chain of events begins to happen.

5. **Notice edges in movement, sound, or breath.** It is helpful to notice edges in your coma work. In this context, edges occur when the flow of a process suddenly seems to stop. It is as if someone were saying a sentence and stopped midway. For example, a comatose person's hand may wave in the air a number of times but then falls back down again.

For training purposes you can always ask your partner, either during or after the exercise, if he is at an edge. This is the best method of learning that I know. Or, you can go back to the experience and find out if it still wants to express itself. For example, if one of the person's arms rises and then falls again, you might try slowly picking up the arm at the wrist and elbow and noticing whether the person begins the motion again. If so, the movement is still in the body and wants to complete itself. If not, then something else is trying to happen.

In a recent training class, a coma work helper gently tested her partner's hand and suddenly found a lot of resistance. The "comatose" person pulled away strongly. They struggled together intensely for about a minute, with locked arms and tension in the "comatose" person's jaw. Then the "comatose" person suddenly relaxed. Her arm flopped down, and she seemed to be at ease. However, if you observed closely, you could see that her jaw was still subtly clenched. When her

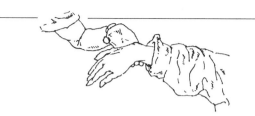

partner tried to pick up her arm again, the same tension resumed and together they were able to complete the struggle she was in the middle of. The "comatose" person had gotten to an edge with her resistance. Afterwards, she said that she wanted very much to continue wrestling but was at an edge and needed her partner's assistance to complete it.

Edges can happen in every channel and are too numerous to mention here.[3] Someone may begin to describe an image and then stop. Feelings may arise and then be disregarded. An important edge to notice in your work with comatose people is found in breathing. For example, a person may make a series of short breaths and then suddenly take a very big breath, then return again to short breaths. You might say, *"Oh, a big breath. That was important. Maybe it will come back, maybe not."*

6. **Don't get stuck.** If you feel that nothing is happening, it is probably time to try another approach. Notice the person's signals and posture, and try other methods. Don't get stuck on one thing that isn't working. Feel free to try new methods. (When you are with a comatose person and you consistently do not receive much feedback, take a break, relax, and come back later.)

7. **Use your intuition, and notice feedback.** While it is most helpful to use blank-access techniques and not to project your own ideas about what is happening onto someone in a coma, in this instance you will try to catch your fantasies or intuitions about what the person is experiencing and verbalize them. As mentioned earlier, some people find that they fall into a light trance state accompanied by dreamlike images when they are working with a comatose person. These fantasies arise in part from the kinds of signals you are receiving from the comatose person and in part from your own inner process and intuition. Suggest these images or intuitions to your partner using words or short phrases like:

"Mmmm, Love, LIFE!"

"Yes, fight for what you want."

"That looks like a peak experience!"

"What an amazing journey."

Most important, watch for feedback. If it is positive, continue. If you do not receive any feedback, do not continue with your fantasy but continue instead with blank-access interventions.

8. **If feedback is positive, amplify verbally.** If you receive positive feedback to your intuitions—the person responds to a particular word or phrase—verbally amplify them. For example, if the person responds to the word "freedom", continue to speak about freedom, such as by saying:

"Yes, freedom, letting go, no boundaries... so free!"

Use your poetic, mythic abilities to speak or sing to the person about her experience. For example:

A coma helper reported that the comatose person seemed to react strongly to close contact. We imagined that the woman enjoyed being loved and that she wanted to be nurtured and cared for. We told the coma helper to try saying things having to do with love and closeness. We also told the coma helper to talk about her happiness and interest in being with the comatose woman. We encouraged the helper to say something like:

"You love LOVE! It's wonderful to be with you here... what a pleasure to be here and be so close with you!"

In this instance, the woman responded positively, moving her head very close to the helper and beginning to make sounds in response to the helper's words.

It is difficult to teach this aspect of the work. Your own experience as well as feedback from your partner will be your best teacher.

Remember to tell your partner when she has five minutes left to complete her experience before sitting up and giving feedback.

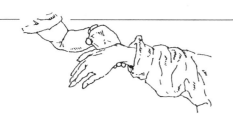

9. **Discuss.** Afterwards, discuss the following with your partner:

❖ For the person lying down:

- What were your experiences?
- Do these experiences connect in any way to your daily life?
- Did the helper mirror and unfold your experiences in a useful way?
- Were the helper's intuitions, words, and songs helpful in unfolding your process?
- What might have been even more helpful?

❖ For the helper:

- What intuitions and fantasies did you have about the person's inner experiences? Use this learning situation to check out the impact of your fantasies on your partner. How close were you to the person's inner experience?
- How comfortable did you feel in assisting your partner with sound, touch, and movement?
- What do you feel you are good at in coma work, and what would you like to practice more? Get feedback, as well, from your partner.
- Did you use binary communication methods? How did that go?

10. **Take notes.** Both people should take time to write in their personal logs about experiences and learning.

Unfolding, Edges, and Intuition

Quick Review

1. Partner lies down.
2. Notice signals, and respond.
3. Test body parts, and notice responses.
4. Unfold.
5. Notice edges in movement, sound, or breath.
6. Don't get stuck.
7. Use your intuition, and notice feedback.
8. If feedback is positive, amplify verbally.
9. Discuss.
10. Take notes.

Exercise 8

Studying a Videotape

It is helpful to videotape participants working with one another and, later, perhaps in the next class session, to study parts of this videotape. Do this periodically throughout your studies to gain more insight into your work and observational skills.

Videotape one of the exercises in which one person acts as if she were in a coma while the helper works with her. To begin with, go around the room and videotape the various people lying on the floor as if they were in a coma. Then videotape various moments when the helpers are working with their partners.

Here are some guidelines for studying the videotape.

Instructions *(all together as a group; 20 to 30 minutes)*

1. **Talk about seeing yourself on video.** Many people are shy to see themselves on video. Sometimes it is startling to see how you look on videotape and that much more startling to see yourself in a "coma-tose" state! So, take time to talk about this first. Get agreement from everyone to watch the tape. Then, as you look at the tape, stop period-ically to find out how people are feeling about viewing themselves.

2. **Discuss what you can learn.** Before you look at the tape, discuss what you hope to learn from watching the video. What elements of coma work will you look for? Some possible answers: observe body pos-tures, notice minimal cues, notice how the coma helper interacts with the comatose person, observe feedback.

3. **Look at the first few minutes.** Show a few minutes of the tape in which people are simply lying down as if they are in a comatose state. Just look. Take in the feeling atmosphere around each person. Allow yourself the freedom to guess, to imagine the "comatose" person's inner experience. Feel or intuit with your sentience what each person may be experiencing. You might physically "assume" these different postures and feel where they are trying to go and what they are trying to express.

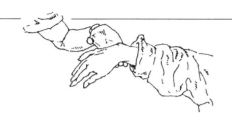

4. **Play again, and describe signals.** Now look at the same part of the tape again. What signals do you see? Notice posture, position of limbs, facial expressions, hair, and so forth. Describe these in sensory-grounded terms. Be exact in your observation. Now what do you see if you do not take anything for granted? (If you need help, review some of the postural signals mentioned in Chapter 9, Exercises 1 and 2.)

5. **Try to connect intuition with signals.** Try to connect your intuitions in step 3 with the exact sensory grounded signals in step 4. Do these signals in any way support your intuitions?

6. **Ask the "comatose" person about her experience.** Now ask the person who was in the "coma" what kind of inner experience she was having. Compare with your guesses. How close were you?

7. **Watch further, and learn from one another.** Watch the tape further. Use this as a great opportunity to learn from one another as much as you can. Watch the coma helper interact with her partner. What do you notice?

Remember to use your sensitivity when you give feedback to one another, knowing that all of us are learning and growing in this area together. Talk to the helper about his experiences. Did he feel comfortable? Awkward? What signals or intuitions was he following?

Notice the following: Does the helper get close? What kinds of feedback does he get to his interventions? Does the "comatose" person take a big breath when the helper is on track? Are there signals that the helper does not see? Do you notice if the "comatose" person gets to an edge?

What metaskills does the coma helper have? In what ways is the helper gifted? Is there anything the helper could do that would be even more useful?

What advice and feedback does the "comatose" person have for the helper? What bodywork methods or metaskills would help the process unfold even further, or did the helper work perfectly? Learn from and teach one another from your inner experiences.

8. **Take notes on learning.** Everyone should write down learning they gained from watching the tape and brainstorming with one another.

Studying a Videotape

Quick Review

1. **Talk about seeing yourself on video.**
2. **Discuss what you can learn.**
3. **Look at the first few minutes.**
4. **Play again, and describe signals.**
5. **Try to connect intuition with signals.**
6. **Ask the "comatose" person about her experience.**
7. **Watch further, and learn from one another.**
8. **Take notes on learning.**

Summary of Learning from Chapter 11

❖ Develop greater ease and more dexterity in your coma work by learning general movement and bodywork techniques.

❖ Learn to sculpt by using your hands like a sensitive potter to contact the body's dreaming process.

❖ Learn to use your hands sentiently to get in touch with processes happening in the musculature of the face and the body.

❖ Use your touch as an open suggestion to which the person responds with her own body process.

❖ Expand your movement abilities by learning a variety of movement amplification techniques.

❖ Discover natural body connections by experimenting alone with movement, breath, and sound.

❖ Acquire an inner feeling for the moment when the process begins to naturally unfold. You will feel on track and that the comatose person's process is flowing naturally.

❖ Try to notice edges in your work.

❖ Practice all coma work techniques learned until this point in a fluid way.

❖ Catch your fantasies and intuitions, and say them. If you get positive feedback, continue with your intuitions. If you get negative feedback, drop what you are imagining and return to blank-access statements and methods.

❖ Study videotapes of your work and learn from your intuition, observational skills, and feedback from classmates.

Notes

1. See my "Hidden Dance: Working with Movement in Process-Oriented Psychology," for a more in-depth discussion of process-oriented movement techniques.

2. There are numerous bodywork and movement techniques that facilitate the experience of somatic congruency. Discussing these is beyond the scope of this book. The reader is referred to such books as Andrea Olsen's *Body Stories*, Blandine Calais-Germain's *Anatomy of Movement*, Aminah Raheem's *Process Acupressure*, and Fritz Smith's *Inner Bridges: Zero Balancing*, as well as general anatomy and physiology books. *The Anatomy Coloring Book* by Kapit, Wynn, and Elson provides excellent pictures that give you the sense of the muscular and skeletal connections.

3. See Arnold Mindell's *Working With the Dreaming Body.*

I n the following exercises you will learn special methods for working with people in comas attributable to brain injury. In addition, to feel your way more fully into the person's world, you will try personal experiments that help you gain a glimpse of what it might be like to be brain injured.

Most of us take our inner body connections for granted. Yet, the seamless connection between parts of our body, which enables us to talk, express ourselves with our hands, or walk, may be disturbed in brain-injured comatose persons. Depending on the site of brain injury, different difficulties of coordination, speech, paralysis, or movement may occur. If the person has had a stroke, one hand may be pulled up toward the chest and in a spasm. The person may be paralyzed on one side. He may have trouble connecting mouth movements to the hands, or he may have an inability to make sounds or formulate words when trying to speak.

When you work with people who are in metabolic comas, they often come out of the coma and relate in ordinary ways, with words. A person in a structural coma, however, may not have the inner body connections to do this. Therefore communication relies in great part on your ability to communicate through fundamental body expressions such as sound, movement, breath, expressions of the mouth, eyes, and forehead, and your ability to get in contact with sentient experiences.

Brain-injured individuals who begin to re-enter ordinary reality are often frustrated by the inability to express themselves fully as they once

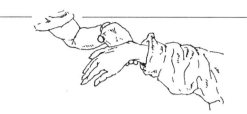

did. Some people who have experienced brain injury may have their full mental abilities intact, yet are not able to get their mouth, hand, or another body part to follow in chorus.

When a brain injury occurs in which there is paralysis or injury to particular parts or areas of the body, there are two basic processes happening simultaneously. One of these processes is connected to the unimpaired part of the body. This part of the body can "re-educate" the other, injured side. The focus is on reconnecting and rehabilitating the parts of the body whose connections have been severed. This focus helps the person relearn coordinated expression.

The other process in brain injury has to do with the side of the body that is paralyzed. Here we find a process of disconnection and dreaming. The injured or paralyzed body part may be completely relaxed and involved in dreaming, which is related to the person's altered-state experiences. Special methods help us discover and unfold the dreaming experiences of that part or side of the body. We have found, paradoxically, that appreciating the experiences of the paralyzed or impaired side of the body helps with the overall recuperation process. When non-ordinary movements—dreaming experiences—are validated, they do not have to disrupt the body but, instead, tend to generate overall recuperation.

Assisting someone in a coma resulting from structural brain injury requires all of the foregoing skills and metaskills plus some special techniques, which include the following:

❖ Reconnecting body parts that are difficult to link because of brain damage.

❖ Accessing processes the comatose person may be able to imagine in fantasy but does not yet have the motor apparatus to express.

❖ Working with fundamental communication modalities including movement, sound, and breath, as well as following sentient tendencies in the body.

- Assisting with the body's natural healing process by helping the unimpaired side or part of the body teach the injured side.

- Discovering and unfolding the dreaming nature of the parts of the body that are impaired.

Metaskills and Teamwork

As mentioned previously, working with structurally brain-injured individuals often takes more time and requires more patience than working with people who have comas of metabolic origins. You need to know from the outset that it is normal for these processes to take time; feedback may also be more subtle. As the helper, you will need encouragement, love, and support.

It is especially helpful—and sometimes crucial when structural comas are involved—to work with at least one other person, both for emotional support and to physically work with the various parts of the body that one person cannot reach alone. As with all previous methods, it is also helpful to teach family members these coma skills so that they can carry on the work when you are not there.

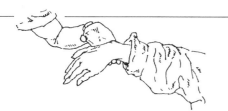

Exercise 1

Working with Facial Communication

Until now, we have worked with communication in terms of the breath, sounds, and movements of the limbs and have experimented with sculpting the face. Here, we will go deeper into specific methods for assisting the experiences happening in the face, including the mouth, the eyelids, and the lips.

Instructions *(in pairs; 5 minutes for exercise, 5 minutes for discussion; then switch)*

1. **Recall learnings.** Discuss with your partner learnings you gained from Exercise 2 in Chapter 11. Together, turn to Chapter 5, Exercise 2 (steps 2 and 3), and study techniques for working with the face, cheeks, jaw, eyes, or brow.

2. **Partner lies down on the floor.** Your partner should lie down on the floor and let himself imagine drifting into a trance state. Sit next to him.

3. **Use sculpting methods with the face.** Begin by adjusting yourself inwardly to your partner's state of consciousness, getting in contact with your own sentient feeling.

   Now use your hands sensitively to sculpt your partner's face. Use any of the methods you have learned, and follow your own sentient experience. Start unobtrusively by touching the person's head or forehead. Continue to use sculpting methods, and access any experiences happening in the facial muscles.

4. **Notice feedback, and mirror it.** Respond to any feedback in the facial muscles with your hands and with sounds or words.

5. **Discuss.** Discuss your experience, and get feedback from your partner.

Working with Facial Communication

Quick Review

1. **Recall learnings.**
2. **Partner lies down on the floor.**
3. **Use sculpting methods with the face.**
4. **Notice feedback, and mirror it.**
5. **Discuss.**

Exercise 2

Personal Experiment: What Is It Like to Be Brain Injured?

One of the best ways I have found to learn about the experience of brain-injured people is to feel what it *may* be like to have a brain injury; to try to know this experience "from the inside out." Recall once again the analogy of someone with a brain injury as the driver of a car in which some of the wires of the car are disconnected. The person attempts to turn the steering wheel, but the tires do not move correspondingly.

Here, you will need to get in contact with the sentient essence of the experience, that is, the very origin of the movement even before it manifests outwardly, because the person may not be able to express her experience in more overt ways. You may be surprised that the sentient origins of experiences can vary greatly from one individual to the next!

Instructions. *(15 minutes; one person guides others through exercise)*

1. **Sit in a comfortable position.**

2. **Imagine experiences.** Try the following thought experiments:

❖ Imagine that you want to walk to the door. You intend to move, but your legs do not respond. Notice what this feels like. Now, use your inner sensing to notice where the impulse to walk originates. The initial impulse can be located at different points for different people.

Possible responses follow. The impulse begins in:

  ▫ My thighs, which have a slight tendency to tighten.
  ▫ My eyes, which start to look in the direction of the door.

❖ Imagine that you see a balloon, which is rising up in front of you. You want to reach for it, but you are unable to. Your arms don't move either because you are heavily drugged, because your body is reduced from metabolic experiences, or because of disruptions caused by brain injury, or a combination of these. What is this experience like? Where does the impulse to reach up originate?

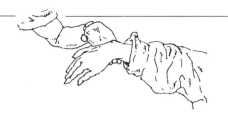

Possible responses follow. The impulse begins in:

- My eyebrows, which want to rise slightly.
- A slight motion of my finger.
- A slight tendency in my shoulders.

❖ Imagine that someone comes into the room. You want to speak to that person. Your mouth begins to move, but no words come out. Where does the impulse to speak begin?

Possible responses follow. The impulse begins in:

- The center of my chest, just as I begin to take a breath.
- Deep inside my throat.
- In my eyes.
- In my cheeks.

❖ Imagine that someone is standing on your right side and is speaking to you. You want to turn your head, but you are unable to move your neck muscles.

Possible responses follow: The impulse starts in:

- A line down the side of my torso.
- The left side of the neck.
- In the twitch of my mouth.
- In my eyes, which want to move to the side.
- In my head, which moved internally without actually moving.

❖ Imagine that you want to reach out to someone and hug them, but only one arm can do that because you are paralyzed on one side. Where does the impulse to hug begin in the paralyzed arm?

3. **Discuss.** Talk about your experiences with the whole group.

Personal Experiment: What Is It Like to Be Brain Injured?

Quick Review

1. Sit in a comfortable position.
2. Imagine experiences.
3. Discuss.

Exercise 3

Brain Injury: Sentient Origins of Experience

When we work with people in coma, we follow either overt signals—such as movements we can see or sounds we can hear—or sentient tendencies before they manifest outwardly. In the following exercise we focus on connecting to sentient experiences. Exercise 5 focuses on both kinds of signals.

Again, a brain-injured comatose person may not have the motor apparatus to express herself outwardly but may feel the sentient beginnings of experiences in her body. She may experience tendencies or impulses which, because of organic problems, cannot rise to the surface in outer expression. The following exercise helps caretakers become more attuned to their partner's sentient experiences.

Instructions. *(in pairs; 15 minutes for one person. Switch, then 10 minutes for group discussion)*

1. **Choose one action.** One of the two people in your dyad should choose one of the following experiences without telling her partner.

   ❖ You want to sit up, but you don't have the ability to do that.

   ❖ You want to walk across the room, but your legs do not move.

   ❖ You want to reach out and hug someone, but only one arm moves slightly. The other is paralyzed.

   ❖ You hear a sound to the right of your right ear. You want to turn toward it but can't quite move your head.

   ❖ Someone approaches. You want to speak to that person, but you are unable to make sounds.

   ❖ You want to turn on your side but can't. You begin, but you are unable to do so.

2. **Lie down, and imagine this experience.** The partner who chose an experience should lie on the floor, start to imagine this experience, and allow it to influence her body.

3. **Helper tries to discover process.** The helper's job is to try to discover which experience the person is having. Don't worry about getting it right! Use this exercise simply to experiment.

   Begin by getting close, pacing the breath, and then using any techniques and skills you have learned until this point. Observe signals, use your hands sentiently, test the limbs, and so forth. You may simply notice a very subtle tensing of a muscle. From this information try to guess the experience the "comatose" person is having.

4. **Help the process unfold.** Help the process unfold. It might help to imagine that you, as the helper, are having this experience. Feel from the inside what would be most helpful to your partner.

   Use sounds, words, and hands-on amplification methods. For example, if you feel one of the person's thigh muscles tensing and you imagine that the person is trying to walk, you can place your hand gently where the muscle is tensing and encourage the person verbally by saying:

   "Go all the way, you'll get there, yes, go...!"

   You can also try to lift the leg, noticing physical responses.

   If you feel that the person's head is trying to move to the right, use your hands where you imagine this movement originating and assist the neck and head in this direction.

5. **If you are lost, get help.** If you, as the helper, feel you cannot discover the process, ask your partner for help. She should instruct you as to what she is experiencing and needing. Then continue to amplify and unfold.

6. **Get feedback.** Take time for your partner to give you feedback about your work. Learn as much as you can from one another about sentient impulses and how to access inner processes.

7. **Collect ideas.** Sit together as a group and collect ideas. If a few of the "comatose" people chose the same experience, did their initial sentient impulses originate in the same or different places? Educate one another about your experiences.

> **Note:** Your coma work may evolve into large-scale or very small-scale interactions. Large-scale interventions may include moving the limbs in an expansive way. Small-scale interventions include minute, subtle interactions such as connecting the upward movement of the eyes with a gentle lifting of the eyebrows. Or you might gently touch the origin of a signal in the body and simply encourage the person to follow her inner experiences there. Remember that for someone in a coma, the most minimal, subtle interactions can be very powerful and meaningful! Most important, follow the process and feedback of the person you are working with.

> *Brain Injury: Sentient Origins of Experience*
>
> **Quick Review**
> 1. Choose one action.
> 2. Lie down, and begin to feel this experience.
> 3. Helper tries to discover process.
> 4. Help the process unfold.
> 5. If you are lost, get help.
> 6. Get feedback.
> 7. Collect ideas.

Exercise 4

Facilitating Coordinated Movement

To facilitate an individual's ability to express herself as fully as possible, it is important to help her rediscover internal connections she may not be able to make because of brain injury. In this exercise, experiment with finding inner body connections in your partner, as you did with yourself in Chapter 11, Exercises 5 and 6.

This kind of work is best done with co-helpers. When you work with more than one person, you can connect distant parts of the body to one another. Also, the more eyes you have, the more you will be able to notice.

Instructions (*This exercise should be done with at least three people; four is best. Take 5 minutes for experimenting with each person, 5 minutes for each discussion.*)

1. **Study together.** As a team, study methods described in Chapter 6, Exercise 1.

2. **One person lies down.** Now one person should lie down while the others sit nearby.

3. **Make a movement.** The person lying down should make a very simple movement such as slightly lifting an arm or a leg, turning the head, arching the back, or taking a big breath.

4. **Respond and amplify.** The helpers should use encouraging sounds and hands-on techniques to amplify this movement.

5. **Helpers discover body connections.** Working as a team, helpers should imagine which body parts and muscle groups connect congruently to this original movement. Imagine which other areas of the body would move congruently with this part. Using your hands, experiment with congruently coordinating the original movement with the movement of other body parts. Move one body part, then progressively add others.

6. **Person on floor notices signals.** The person on the floor should notice internal, subtle signals indicating what would feel most connective

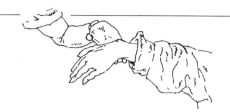

and congruent and then give verbal feedback to the helpers as they are working. Helpers respond by adjusting to this feedback, if necessary.

7. **Discuss.** Discuss this experience with your small group.

8. **Try again.** Repeat steps 1 through 7 with a different person lying on the floor.

Facilitating Coordinated Movement

Quick Review

1. **Study together.**
2. **One person lies down.**
3. **Make a movement.**
4. **Respond and amplify.**
5. **Helpers discover body connections.**
6. **Person on floor notices signals.**
7. **Discuss.**
8. **Try again.**

Exercise 5

Working as a Team: Breath, Movement, and Sound

Now let's try connecting breath, movement, and sound when working with others. This exercise is best done with two or more co-helpers. Following the exercise I have included a transcription of a supervision session illustrating some of these methods.

Instructions *(groups of three or four; 20 minutes for practice; 15 minutes for discussion)*

1. **Review methods.** As a team, turn to Chapter 6, Exercise 2 (step 5), and review methods.

2. **One person lies down on the floor.** One person in the group lies down on the floor and imagines that he is in a trance or comatose state.

3. **As a team, approach and follow breathing and signals.** One helper should approach the person, following the breath and gently taking hold of the wrist. If there are no other outstanding signals, all helpers should join in pacing the breathing and adding by gently holding the other wrist, a foot, and the head. (See Chapter 4, Exercise 1, for details.)

    As a group, try to follow and respond to minimal cues, using movement and sound to amplify signals. Once you have begun to work with other signals, you no longer have to pace the breath. The idea is to coordinate your work together in order to follow the person's process and congruently help it unfold, not to do many different methods at once. Amplify overall body posture, test body parts, and respond to any feedback. Take time. Let each signal and interaction have time to unfold before jumping to the next.

    Don't be afraid to talk to your teammates as you work, in case you notice a new signal or want to move around to coordinate your work. The comatose person will be helped most by the fluid coordination and sensitivity of your group.

4. **Notice the strongest signal, amplify it, and make connections in other parts of the body.** Notice the body area where you get the most energetic signal or feedback—either an overt or a sentient signal. As a

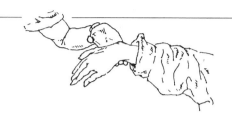

team, try to connect this experience to sound, breath, and movement in other parts of the body.

5. **Notice feedback, and unfold.** Use your collective feelings as a group to know when you are on track.

6. **Discuss.** Discuss your experiences.

❖ For the person lying down:

▫ What was it like to have more than one helper working with you?

▫ How did you experience the helpers' attempt to connect your movement, breath, and sound?

▫ Is there any constructive advice you would give them about following your process and your sense of congruency?

❖ For the helpers:

▫ What was it like for you to work as a team? Was it difficult to coordinate your work together? Did you feel comfortable? Awkward? Shy? Better or worse than when working alone?

▫ Was it difficult or easy as a team to develop congruency in movement, sound, and breath in the "comatose" person?

▫ Could you sense as a group when the person's process was unfolding?

7. **Take notes.** Record your experiences in your personal log.

Working as a Team: Breath, Movement, and Sound

Quick Review

1. Review methods.
2. One person lies down on the floor.
3. As a team, approach and follow breathing and signals.
4. Notice the strongest signal, amplify it, and make connections in other parts of the body.
5. Notice any feedback, and unfold.
6. Discuss.
7. Take notes.

Supervision Example

The following description of a coma supervision given by Arny and myself to three coma workers via telephone may give you more insight into aspects of the previous exercises. The coma work helpers were at the bedside of "Cindy," the comatose person; they had been visiting her for quite some time and had already established intimate contact.

Cindy was breathing at a normal rate. We recommended that one helper put her hand on Cindy's stomach and pace her breath.

Then we suggested that the same helper put two fingers of the other hand gently between Cindy's teeth. Each time she inhaled, the helper was to try to open her mouth a little bit, alternately pressing on the stomach as she exhaled.

The helper reported that Cindy bit slightly on her fingers and began to make sounds and movements as if she were eating something. We recommended that the helper follow by saying, "*Yes, go ahead, we see your mouth ... hmmm ... speak more if you like.*"

We then suggested that another helper stand behind Cindy; every time she made a noise, the helper was to press gently on the muscles of the back of the neck. Cindy began to make more sounds.

We then suggested that everyone make sounds together whenever Cindy made a sound. Cindy made very strong and exciting sounds like, "Whoooah!" We then recommended that the helpers accompany her by making more sounds and saying words like, "*Life!*" and "*Love!*"

This shows how to connect breath, mouth movements, and sound.

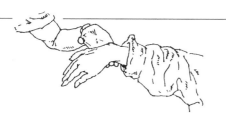

Exercise 6

Personal Experiment: What Is It Like to Be Paralyzed?

Paralysis or injury of one part or side of the body is common in coma resulting from brain injury. To gain a better sense of this experience, let's try to feel our way into what it is like to be paralyzed. In Exercise 7 we explore special methods for working with others. In this Exercise, for ease in description, I call one side of the body "unimpaired" and the other side "paralyzed."

Instructions: *(10 minutes; one person guiding others through the exercise)*

1. **Lie down.** Find a comfortable position lying on the floor.

2. **Make motions with both arms.** Move both of your arms as you like.

3. **Imagine paralysis on one side.** Now, imagine that one arm is injured or paralyzed while the other is not. Choose either hand to be paralyzed. Just feel this experience for a moment.

4. **Make a few motions with the "unimpaired" arm.** Make any motions you like with the "unimpaired" arm. Do you notice any sensations at the same time in the "paralyzed" arm?

   Ordinarily, both arms move together in tandem. Feel the impulse for both arms to move together. This experience helps you know from the inside how you might help someone get in touch with the origins of movements, which in turn assists you in your knowledge of reconnecting the unified movement of the arms.

5. **Imagine the "unimpaired" arm as parent.** Now imagine that the "unimpaired" arm is like a good parent and that it could "baby" the "paralyzed" arm. Feel how it might do that in any way you like, such as stroking the "injured" arm, moving it about, or the like.

6. **Make movement with the "unimpaired" arm, and let it help the other arm do this as well.** Now make any movement with the "unimpaired" arm, such as reaching out. Begin again, this time helping the "unimpaired" hand and arm grasp the "paralyzed" arm. Guide the "paralyzed" arm as both arms make the same motion together (Figure 71).

7. **Guide "paralyzed" arm to the face.** Now use your "unimpaired" arm and hand to grasp your "paralyzed" hand. Guide the paralyzed hand and fingers to your face, and help the fingers gently caress your mouth, nose, eyelids, and forehead (Figure 72). As you do this, say:

"My "right" (unimpaired) hand is teaching my "left" (paralyzed) hand about my face. These are my lips, and now these are my eyes, my nose [and so forth] … My right hand is teaching this to my left."

8. **Discuss.** Discuss this experience with another class member.

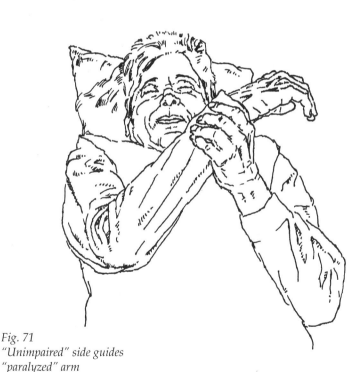

Fig. 71
"Unimpaired" side guides "paralyzed" arm

Fig. 72
"Unimpaired" side guides "paralyzed" hand and fingers to the face

---

Personal Experiment: What Is It Like to Be Paralyzed?

Quick Review

1. Lie down.
2. Make motions with both arms.
3. Imagine paralysis on one side.
4. Make a few motions with the "unimpaired" arm.
5. Imagine the "unimpaired" arm as parent.
6. Make movement with the "unimpaired" arm, and let it help other arm do this as well.
7. Guide "paralyzed" arm to face.
8. Discuss.

Work with Brain Injury | 233

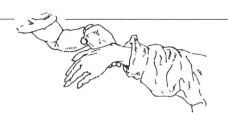

Exercise 7

One Side Teaches the Other and Following the Dreaming Body

The following exercise is helpful when one part or side of the body is injured or paralyzed as a result of structural brain injury. Again, there are two parts to the paralysis experience. One part has to do with striving toward recuperation, and the other part has to do with unfolding the dreaming process.

Support both aspects of the process. At one point, encourage the part of the body that is not paralyzed to re-educate and rehabilitate the impaired part of the body. At another point, encourage the person to follow the experiences occurring in the paralyzed or injured side or part of the body.

Which process you follow depends on feedback. Try one method. If you receive strong feedback, stay with it. If not, try the other method. This may change within one session or over time. The following exercise explores both methods.

Instructions *(in pairs, 5 minutes per person; 5 minutes for feedback)*

1. **Partner imagines one side paralyzed.** One partner should imagine that one of his arms is impaired or paralyzed.

2. **Helper tries methods.** Experiment with the methods described in Chapter 6, Exercise 3.

3. **Notice any feedback, and encourage.** Use sound and touch to assist your partner.

4. **Discuss.** Gain feedback from your partner about your work.

One Side Teaches the Other and Following the Dreaming Body

Quick Review

1. Partner imagines one side paralyzed.
2. Helper tries methods.
3. Notice any feedback, and encourage.
4. Discuss.

Summary of Learning from Chapter 12

❖ Working with people who have had structural brain injury requires time, patience, and knowledge of fundamental body communication.

❖ Work with basic communication centers, including the breath, the eyes, sounds, and movements of the limbs, as well as the mouth, the eyelids, and the lips.

❖ Facilitate congruency by helping the whole body express itself as an integrated unit. Notice what signals the person is making. Use your skills to connect these signals to other body areas in a fluid way.

❖ Learn how to work as a team to connect movement, sound, touch, and breath.

❖ When one part or side of the body is injured or paralyzed, there are two processes at hand. One process has to do with re-education, and the other follows the dreaming process of the body. Facilitate both processes.

❖ Help the unimpaired side of the body re-educate the impaired side, and help the impaired or paralyzed side of the body express its dreaming process.

❖ In all cases, watch the feedback to determine the direction of your interactions.

Chapter 13

I n this chapter we will learn methods that are useful during the rehabilitative process when the comatose person is emerging from coma into a more wakeful state.[1] We will apply more general process work methods because the person is ready for these therapeutic body- and movement-oriented interventions.

The exercises apply to people who seem close to the surface, who respond easily to simple communication, and with whom you have good response and feedback. They may, however, have physical impairments that hamper rehabilitation in such areas as speech, cognition, memory, and motor coordination.

Many of these people experience the frustration of not being able to express themselves or use their bodies as they once did. For example, one young woman, who recuperated from brain injury and was beginning to re-enter high school, was frustrated because one of her hands was still somewhat lame. She said that she would tell her hand to write something but it would move very slowly.

As mentioned in Chapter 1, coma and its various stages of recovery can be viewed as spanning a continuum from the deepest trance state—where the person is very far away from ordinary reality—to the other end of the spectrum, in which people are closer to ordinary states of consciousness and are more able to adapt to everyday reality.

When you work with someone who is recuperating from brain injury after a coma, most likely you will find him straddling these two worlds.

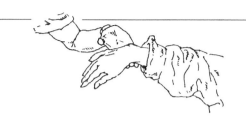

While parts of the person are reaching toward everyday life, other aspects of him lag behind and remain in a kind of dreamy inner state. The person may fluctuate back and forth between a more wakeful and a more dreamy type of awareness.

Therefore working with people in coma rehabilitation requires the ability to work in both worlds. Just as we practiced with the exercise on paralysis in Chapter 11, we need to value both of these processes. Which process you focus on, of course, depends on the feedback you receive. If someone is yearning for and tending toward more connection in everyday life and recuperation, this is the direction. If the person is in a dreamy state and does not relate to everyday reality, or is interested in exploring his trancelike experiences, this becomes the focus. In such cases, you can use any of the skills learned until this point.

Recall the man mentioned in Chapter 1, who was out of his coma but who continually talked about music. His helpers stressed that he know the current date and time. They were hoping for even steadier recollection of his ordinary cognitive abilities. However, his lack of responding to commands indicated that he was still in a "dreaming" state. As mentioned in Chapter 12, we have found that if these dreaming experiences are appreciated, recuperation is hastened. People feel validated, and their dreaming processes do not have to disrupt their lives.

While this "straddling of worlds" is distinct in people recovering from brain injury, the flow between deep inner states and ordinary life is often apparent even in the deepest coma. Some of these people seem immersed in inner experiences and do not seem to want to adapt to ordinary life. Sometimes, however, they reach across to the everyday world, relate to you and your questions, or come out of the coma. Recall Peter, mentioned in Chapter 1. He was in a very deep coma, came out of it, talked with us, and then returned to his inner state. Some people near death awaken, some express their feelings to their family, and some return fully to ordinary life, whereas others are immersed in their dreaming, inner experiences. (See the example in Chapter 16.)

Exercise 1

Inner Work: Body Scan and Congruence

The following exercise addresses both the tendency toward entering everyday life and the tendency to dream.

In this exercise you experiment alone with yourself. In Exercise 2 you will practice with a partner.

Instructions *(guided by one person, 10 minutes all together)*

1. **Lie down.** Lie down on the floor and get comfortable. Take a minute to relax and be with yourself.

2. **Do body scan.** Do a body scan, beginning with your head and moving down to your toes. (The person leading this exercise should tell everyone to bring their awareness to the tops of their head, their skull, the eyes and face, and proceed by guiding class members' awareness all the way down the body.)

3. **Notice where process is happening.** Now, go back over your body and sense where "process" is happening in the strongest way. Where is something trying to happen? Notice how much energy is in this part of the body. Is there a lot or just a little?

   The word *process* here refers to energy. It is purposefully vague so that you can fill in your own understanding of this word and sense your own inner energies.

4. **Feel and amplify.** Feel this part of your body. Begin to amplify the sensation you have there: make it a bit stronger. Now amplify it by spreading it out and feeling the same energy or quality in different parts of your body until you experience it in your whole body. Add breath, sound, and movement—a lot or a little depending on the amount of energy you experienced originally—which mirror this feeling to amplify it further.

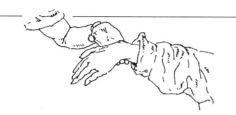

5. **Make an image.** Make a picture of that experience, and continue to unfold the experience with images, sounds, movements, and breath.

6. **Use mythic words, poetry, or song.** Try to embellish your experience further by expressing it in words, poetry, or song. Write it down or sing a song to yourself.

7. **Share your experience with a partner and answer questions.**

❖ Where did you initially feel the strongest process in your body?

❖ How open were you to exploring this?

❖ Were you able to amplify this experience throughout your body? Could you use movement, sound, breath, and images to unfold the experience?

❖ Share your poetry or song.

❖ Now ask yourself: Does that experience want to be experienced as it is without having to adapt to ordinary life, or does it want to be integrated into your ordinary everyday reality?

Inner Work: Body Scan and Congruence

Quick Review

1. **Lie down.**
2. **Do body scan.**
3. **Notice where process is happening.**
4. **Feel and amplify.**
5. **Make an image.**
6. **Use mythic words, poetry, or song.**
7. **Share your experience with a partner and answer questions.**

Exercise 2

Following Inner Processes with Body Scan

Now try the previous method with a partner.

Instructions *(in pairs; 15 minutes per person)*

1. **Establish binary communication.** For ease, discuss with your partner ahead of time who will act like a "comatose person-in-recuperation" and which signal she will use for yes-and-no answers. For example, a finger movement may indicate "yes" and no movement of the finger may mean "no." (When you work with a comatose person, you use binary communication methods to establish this signal.)

2. **Lie down and feel body.** The "comatose person" lies down and imagines that she is in a stage of coma in which she is close to the surface but is unable to speak. Encourage the comatose person to take time to feel her body. The helper should make contact with her partner by feeling her way into the person's state and by pacing the breath.

3. **Scan the body and ask where the most process is happening.** After a few minutes, tell your partner, who is lying down, that in a minute you will slowly guide your hands just over her body and ask, "Where do you feel most process in your body? Where do you feel the impulse of life most strongly?"

   Now, as the helper, begin to move your hands about 12 inches above the body, moving them slowly from the head to the feet, saying:

   "My hands are here, over the top of your head, now your face, neck, shoulders [and so forth]... Notice the area where you experience the most process in your body."

   Ask the person lying down to make a signal using her binary method at the spot where process or life energy seems the strongest. Wait for a response.

4. **Ask about amount of energy.** Once you have identified where the person experiences the most life in her body, ask her if there is a lot of energy

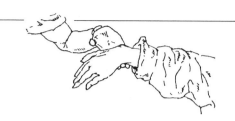

there. Wait for a response. Ask if there is a little energy there. Or ask if there is a medium amount of energy there. Wait for a binary response.

Once you have a response, determine more exactly the amount of energy. Ask such binary questions as:

"Is it enough energy to push a ball? A feather? Is it enough to push a house? A truck? Enough to smile?"

Once you have a response, you will know how much energy the person feels in that area of the body and how much energy is available. If there is a little energy, do not ask the person to do too much. Follow the feedback.

5. **Ask partner to feel energy in other parts of the body.** Now ask your partner if she can make that energy available in other parts of her body by feeling it in various places. Can she feel the same energy in her feet? In her hands? In her chest? Can she use that energy to make a smile? If one of her hands or another part of her body is injured or impaired, can she feel the same energy in that part of the body? Pause after each request, and notice responses.

6. **Unfold energy in fantasy.** Ask your partner if she can transform the feeling of that energy into a visual fantasy. Can she make a picture of that energy? If she can, ask her to watch that image unfold. Let it evolve like a story. Simply encourage her to watch these images for a couple of minutes.

7. **Take a break.** Take a break. Encourage the person to relax.

8. **Discuss.** Discuss your experiences with one another.

Following Inner Processes with Body Scan

Quick Review

1. Establish binary communication.
2. Lie down and feel body.
3. Scan the body, and ask where the most process is happening.
4. Ask about amount of energy.
5. Ask partner to feel energy in other parts of the body.
6. Unfold energy in fantasy.
7. Take a break.
8. Discuss.

Exercise 3

Long-Term Goals

As the comatose person's rehabilitation evolves, it is helpful to ask questions with an eye to his potential re-emergence into everyday life. The following questions help the comatose person consider his attitudes and goals, his motivations and drives toward everyday life. He can contemplate long-term goals and steps toward these aims, and consider the possible meaning of the comatose state for his everyday life.

If the person can be motivated, the recuperation time is shortened. If he cannot be motivated, it is important to find out where he is with his life and to help him lead the kind of life he feels he would like to live. That motivation, even if it's not what the person used to have in his everyday life, can then be tapped and used for recuperation. For example, if someone wants to lead a different kind of life than he used to live, what kind would it be? Direct rehabilitation toward leading that kind of lifestyle.

Instructions *(in pairs; 10 minutes per person)*

1. **Establish binary communication.** Decide ahead of time with your partner who will act like the "comatose" person and which signal he will use to answer yes-and-no questions, such as a finger motion, twitching of an eyebrow, or the like.

2. **Wait, then approach.** Your partner lies down and imagines that he is in a state in which he has had a coma as a result of brain injury but is now beginning to recover. The helper should give him time to feel his way into this experience. Now approach him, and begin to make contact by means of methods learned previously.

3. **Pose questions about long-term goals.** After a few minutes, ask your partner questions about his long-term goals. Some useful questions about these goals are:

"Do you want to live?"

"If so, do you want to be a mother, father?

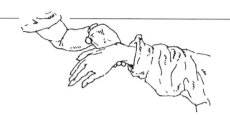

"Do you want to be a student?"

"A teacher?"

"An artist?"

"A therapist?"

"A lover?"

"A business person?"

"A writer?"

"Or a ..."

Use your imagination to ask other questions that might be relevant. When you work with someone in this state, you can use your knowledge of that person and his goals before the coma for ideas, although it is important to include other possibilities in your questions because the person may be feeling different now about the future than he did before the coma.

Ask other questions, such as:

"Are you looking forward to life?"

"Do you want to come all the way back?"

4. **Ask questions about the meaning of the coma.** Ask the person questions about the meaning of his comatose state, such as:

"Was the comatose state a way to relax or go on vacation?"

"A way to get closer to God?"

"An attempt to go inside and get away from the world?"

"To have a love affair?" (Many people in these states have affairs with spirit-like lovers.)

"To enter or complete a mythic battle?"

"To climb a mountain?"

"To be with nature?"

These questions are important because without an understanding of the meaning behind comatose states, inner processes tend to repeat. Once you know the answers to these questions, you can, later, help the person find ways of integrating the meaning of the comatose state in his everyday life.

The person on the floor should imagine what a comatose state could mean for her and respond through binary communication.

5. **Discuss.** Discuss this experience with your partner. The person who was lying down should address the following questions:

❖ What questions were helpful?

❖ What questions would have been more helpful?

❖ What did you learn about yourself?

The helper should discuss her experiences as well.

Long-Term Goals

Quick Review

1. **Establish binary communication.**
2. **Approach the comatose person.**
3. **Pose questions about long-term goals.**
4. **Ask questions about the meaning of the coma.**
5. **Discuss.**

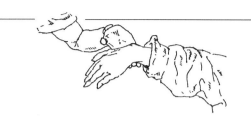

Summary of Learning from Chapter 13

❖ People who are recuperating from coma pass through various stages on a spectrum ranging from the deepest trance state to full recovery and adaptation to ordinary reality.

❖ While working with someone who is the recuperation process from brain injury, most likely you will find her straddling the dreaming world and the ordinary world. Learn to appreciate and work with both experiences depending on the person's feedback.

❖ Learn to identify where process or life energy is happening most strongly in the body, and use it to assist the rest of the body in its recuperation process.

❖ Help the person emerging from coma to consider and prepare for everyday life by asking questions about motivation and goals.

❖ Ask the person about the meaning of her comatose state, and, later, when she is out of the coma, help her to integrate this experience in everyday life.

Note

1. These methods are adapted from Arny Mindell's courses on extreme states and supervision, Portland, Oregon, spring 1997.

T he following questions are intended as a review of your learning. They will help you integrate and absorb some of the information and experiences you have gained throughout your coma work studies. Take time to consider the questions, to consider your personal experiences, and to evaluate your work with others. Write down your answers in detail in your personal log, then discuss them with a partner, or with your whole group (or both).

Exercise 1

Exploring Your Motivation

Remember the first exercise in Chapter 7, in which you answered the question, "Why do this work?" Consider this question again, now that you have completed your learning.

Instructions (*alone; 5 minutes*)

1. **Recall the question "Why do I want to do this work?"** Look back at the answer you initially wrote down to this question.

2. **Consider the question again.** Is there anything you would change or add?

3. **Write down your responses.**

Exploring Your Motivation

Quick Review

1. Recall the question.
2. Consider the question again.
3. Write down your responses.

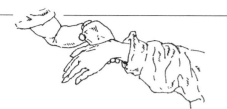

Exercise 2

Personal Questions

Take time to write down thoughts concerning your personal growth and personal experiences.

Instructions *(alone; 10 minutes; then 10 minutes for discussion with a colleague)*

1. **Recall your personal learning.** What have you learned about:

❖ Following your own inner processes?

❖ Your altered states?

❖ Your sentient experiences?

❖ Your feelings about death?

2. **Think about a significant personal experience.** Remember a significant experience you had during an exercise when you were the "comatose" person. Consider the following:

❖ What was important to you about this experience? Why?

❖ Which part of this experience will you remember?

❖ In what ways might this experience affect your everyday life?

3. **Recall learning about personal edges.** What have you learned about:

❖ Your edges in relation to contact, touch, and intimacy?

❖ Your edges concerning the use of sound and movement?

❖ Your edges concerning altered state experiences?

4. **Take notes.** Write your answers in the personal log.

5. **Discuss.** Share your answers with a partner.

Personal Questions

Quick Review

1. **Recall your personal learning.**
2. **Think about a significant personal experience.**
3. **Recall learning about personal edges.**
4. **Take notes.**
5. **Discuss.**

Exercise 3

Integrating Skills and Metaskills

Consider the following questions, which will help you assimilate and integrate some of the learning you have gained about coma work skills and metaskills. First, spend time alone, considering and writing down answers to these questions. Then, to help you integrate some of this information, discuss your answers with a partner.

Instructions *(alone; 15 minutes writing down answers; 20 minutes in discussion with a colleague)*

1. **Review metaskills.**

❖ What metaskills or feeling attitudes are natural to you in working with comatose states?

❖ Which ones are still in the process of developing?

2. **Recall skills.**

❖ Identify central skills you have learned for working with people in comas.

❖ Which skills do you feel most comfortable with?

❖ Which ones would you like to practice further?

❖ Make a list of some of the minimal cues you noticed or learned about.

❖ Describe some methods for amplifying minimal cues.

❖ Describe methods you learned that involve the use of your hands, sound, movement work, and sentient touch.

❖ How do you develop binary communication with a comatose person? How comfortable do you feel with this skill?

❖ How well are you progressing with your ability to use sentient touch?

3. **Review your work with people in comas resulting from brain injury.**

❖ How well are you doing in facilitating congruency in the body by connecting body parts?

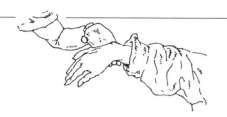

❖ How is your work progressing in respect to communication in terms of the eyes, mouth, and breath?

❖ How are you doing with connecting to the sentient origins of a person's experience?

❖ What do you feel you still need to learn to work as part of a team?

❖ How are you doing with skills oriented toward working with the unimpaired and dreaming sides of the body?

❖ Review learning associated with people who are recuperating and are close to the surface of everyday reality, including:

▫ Discovering and making life energy available to the person's overall process and recuperation.

▫ Exploring the comatose person's long-term goals.

▫ Investigating the potential meaning of the comatose state.

4. **Consider future learning.** How will you continue to develop your coma work skills? Where, when, and with whom?

5. **Talk to a colleague.** Spend some time discussing answers to the previous questions with a co-learner. Help one another fill in gaps in your learning.

Integrating Skills and Metaskills

Quick Review

1. Review metaskills.
2. Recall skills.
3. Review your work with people in structural comas.
4. Consider future learning.
5. Talk to a colleague.

Exercise 4

Group Discussion

As a whole group of learners, spend some time, now, discussing your learnings and future growth and training.

Instructions *(as a whole group, 30 minutes)*

1. **Discuss personal experiences.** Which personal experiences were especially significant to you?

2. **Review skills and metaskills.** Which skills and metaskills have you learned that you would like to remember?

3. **Explore future growth and training.** How will you continue your inner development and outer learning, alone, with a few people, or as a whole group?

4. **Celebrate yourselves.** Celebrate yourselves for learning to penetrate the deepest realm of all human experience! You are true healers because you are also explorers!

Group Discussion

Quick Review

1. Discuss personal experiences.
2. Review skills and metaskills.
3. Explore future growth and training.
4. Celebrate yourselves.

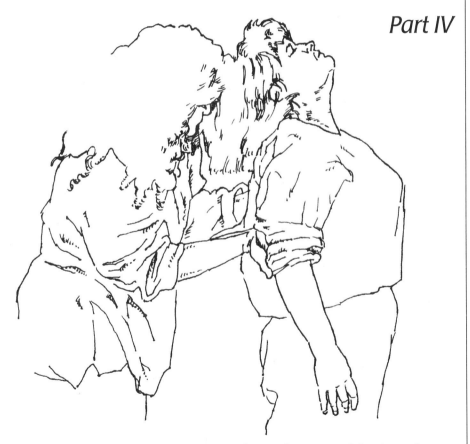

Part IV

Case Histories and Interviews

Follow where people are at—their bodies and their souls will tell you what to do.

The Body Knows Best

Chapter 15

Arnold Mindell

R*ecently, Arny was interviewed on a network television program about his work with people in comatose states. Although only a portion of the interview was aired on the program, I was able to obtain the original taped footage. An edited transcription of his responses follows. Because this was a TV interview, Arny's descriptions are casual and simplified and provide a lively introduction to the development of coma work, as well as a personal chat with him on his feelings about life and death.*

As a Jungian analyst and therapist, I started working with people who had psychosomatic complaints, as well as those who were seriously ill. I worked with these people over long periods of time. Some of them got better; some became seriously ill and were hospitalized. And so I went to the hospitals with them and began to talk with them in all their various stages of consciousness, including comatose states.

This was in Zurich in the 1970s. Each time I went to the hospital to work with a person, families visiting loved ones in comatose states would ask me to work with them.

So I started to work with people I had never met before—on the spot—in contrast to what I had been doing, which was working with people over long periods of time or in brief therapy situations. I suddenly found myself working with people in altered states of consciousness who were either in a partial or persistent vegetative state or comatose and near death.

I had many profound experiences. My name got around Zurich and a lot of people were asking me to work with their relatives and their friends. I had so many incredible, outstanding, unspeakable experiences—yet I promised myself I would never tell anybody about them because I thought that nobody would believe me.

It was a good ten or fifteen years before I said anything to anybody about what I was experiencing. It wasn't until my wife, Amy, began to work with me in the hospitals, and to see the things that actually happened, that I started to talk publicly about what I had been doing. Amy was also witnessing the same things.

In the beginning I saw many people who had incredible awakenings. So many of the people I began to work with would awaken in some form or another, just before dying, and speak about the most wondrous stuff.

Types of Comas and Communication

There are comas resulting from brain injury and near-death comas wherein people dying slowly of either old age or a terminal illness go semi-comatose or fully comatose. Even people who die fairly rapidly will, just before death, go through longer or shorter periods of comatose states wherein they are not arousable. But that doesn't mean they don't want to communicate. It means they don't want to communicate in the style that other people expect them to use. That's one of the big keys to working with people in comas.

I have, to date, never come across anyone in a coma—be it due to severe brain injury, to metabolic problems, or to old age—who hasn't been reachable in some form or other by the kind of communication we do. Everyone can be communicated with, though not everybody gets up and says, "Hello, thank you for talking with me. I want to tell you what I'm thinking." I'm talking about subtle things like color changes in the cheeks.

There are many ways to distinguish different states of consciousness a comatose person enters. People who are in a comatose state prior to death due to metabolic problems may well look asleep, maybe even peaceful. Or they may be slightly agitated so that the body moves in subtle ways. These people, who are close to the surface, can be reached relatively easily in about twenty minutes.

Somebody who has had a severe brain injury is likely to have corticoid or decorticate posturing so that their hands are up like this [Arny puts his hands up near his heart; they are bent at the elbows, the fingers pointing in and downward]. Or if they've had a stroke, one side of the body may be up like this and in a spasm [he raises only one arm]. These people are in vegetative-type comas and are more difficult to reach. You can touch various body parts and they will not show, to the naked eye, any movements whatsoever. You can't work with these people with only verbal methods. And if they come back they may not be able to speak in the way that they did before. So that's a deeper, more vegetative coma.

I have so many examples, but the one that comes to mind just now is one I mention in the beginning of my book *Coma*. I met a man in one of the hospices in Miami, a man in his early eighties who had cancer and had been dying slowly over a long period of time. The man hadn't spoken to anyone for months. I was working in that hospice with somebody else and the nurses asked me if I would spend some time with this man. He would make very loud noises while he was in his coma. He'd roar "whooa" and "wow" and "rhhh" and make all sorts of sounds that disturbed the other patients.

So I went into his room and took a look at this man who was apparently in his last stages of life. He was withdrawn and emaciated, lying stiff as a board in his bed, eyes closed. I walked by the bed and said, "Ooooohh." He responded right away, "Wooooh." I said, "Whooah" and he said, "Woohh." And I thought, well now, that's a kind of communication, so let's go for it. I repeated, "Woohh" and he amplified what I had said by responding, "Woooh, woooooh!" And then I said, "Woooh, weeeeeeeee!"

And there we were in line with one another. Suddenly his eyes opened. At first I saw only the whites of his eyes; he looked way up like this [Arny's eyes look up so that only the whites show] and he said, "Woohooo." From my studies of bodywork and communication, I knew he might be seeing something. "So what are you seeing? Do you see it?" He said, "Do you see it?" I said, "No, I don't quite see it, but just about, what is it?"

He said, "I see a white ship, an all white ship, a white ship." From my work as a therapist I knew I'd better climb into this altered state of consciousness. Let's forget that it's called a coma, and let's forget that he's dying, and let's communicate with him where he's at. I said, "There's a big white ship coming." He said, "And it's coming for me!" And I said, "Wow, are you gonna go?" And he said, "No, not me, I'm not going anywhere." And I said, "That makes sense to me, I wouldn't go if a white ship just pulled up for me either."

He had been stuck in this state for a long time. I thought to myself, he's all excited about seeing this white ship and that's why he was making all those noises that they were calling a disturbance or a coma or whatever. So I said to him, "Whoah! Let's get on that ship and take a look around just for a quick peek." "All right," he said. I added, "Let's check out who's driving it."

I could sense his boarding that white ship and looking around. I could see his eyes rolling back and forth as he said, "Whooo, whoo." I was going with him so I said, "I bet it's wild in there. Who's driving it?" Animatedly he answered, "Whooo, it's angels driving that ship, angels are driving that damn ship!" I said, "That's interesting, that's new for me, I don't think I ever heard of a ship driven by angels. What's down in the boiler room? What kind of a motor has it got?" (Being a physicist, I have to admit I was still interested in motors and things like that!) He went down to the boiler room in his fantasy, looked around and said, "There's angels in that boiler room, too!" "Well," I said, "All right, where's the ship going?" He said, "Wow, that ship is going to Bermuda!" "Woah, Bermuda," I said. He said, "Yeah, that ship's going on vacation."

I said, "What's that ship cost?" He checked it out with the angels. He went downstairs and upstairs and took some time. "What's it cost, what's it cost?" he said. "That ship doesn't cost anything!" "Well, what do you think?" I said and he answered, "Well, I don't know if I can go." "Why not?" I asked. "I've got to get up tomorrow morning at eight and go to work," he said. "Well," I said, "it doesn't cost anything, that ship. You can take a trip on it if you want, or not. If you take the trip maybe I'll meet you there one of these days in Bermuda—and if you don't take the trip, that's fine too."

I never know where people want to go. This work never tells people, "You've got to come back to life" or "You're supposed to die." Many people will come back to life right away, while some people don't.

The last thing I said to Sam was, "OK, you make your choice about if you want to take that free trip or go back to work tomorrow morning. Both are fine with me. See ya." "Yep," he said, "Good-bye." He closed his eyes and went to sleep.

I walked out of the room and went back to my other clients. A few minutes later I came back to check on him. The nurses were standing around him and one exclaimed, "My god, he fell asleep and he died!" And that was the end of his life.

He had been unable to let go and die. He had been stuck in a hospice for months and months. But apparently he made the decision to take that free trip to Bermuda. He had been stuck in an ordinary problem that all of us have at one time or another. He just couldn't decide whether or not to take a vacation. In part, his comatose state reflected his frustration at not knowing what was happening to him and the conflict of being offered this very beautiful trip to Bermuda. For him, that was what a coma was. That's one example of a very vivid coma.

Communication and Ethics

I feel the whole goal of working with people in comas is to connect with them and to incorporate their feedback, their responses to what is happening to them from the medical team and from the family as much as possible.

To my way of thinking, it's not ethically sound that the medical team—which usually has no sense of what the person is going through—or the family—who knew the person in normal states of consciousness but may not have known the person at all in altered states of consciousness—are solely allowed to make decisions about those in a severely altered state of consciousness. That is unethical to me. Yet it is a widespread practice, because people just don't know how to relate to people in comas.

I do understand that the medical community and the family are doing their absolute best. But years from today, people are going to look back at this period of medicine and they are going to say, "My God, wow, the decisions on whether or not to pull the tubes on people in comas were made without asking the people themselves, without even trying to communicate with them."

So the goal is to communicate with people and to incorporate their decisions. You don't have to follow their decisions. Some people may say they want to die. You needn't follow it, but you do need to know what their wishes are. And some may indicate that they want to live, and you need to take those responses seriously also.

When I say "communicate with somebody in a coma," I mean, first of all, remember them the way they used to be, what they used to say. When they weren't in a coma, they said, "Oh well, if I ever get into a vegetative state, forget it, pull the tubes on me." They may not know what it's like to be in a drowsy or deep state. They may think that it's just dreadful or horrible. You need to know that about them. What they say ahead of time is terribly important. You've got to take that into consideration.

You've also got to take the family and the medical community into consideration because sometimes both are burdened with the care of someone who is in a long-term vegetative state, which is very expensive and time-consuming.

When I say "communicate with the person," I also mean getting down with them where they are at in the comatose state, altering your own consciousness, putting your face near their face, speaking gently in their ear about what they're experiencing, saying to them to follow what they are experiencing, to believe in their experiences.

In this kind of work, you have to ask yourself again and again, "What am I doing? What is my job?" Technical problems come in here, existential and ethical problems and questions about the meaning of life come in here. Whose meaning of life? My meaning of life or the other person's meaning of life? This is an important distinction, and there are no permanent answers. The meaning of life and death varies from individual to individual. That is important.

When we can't communicate with a comatose person, the family, the state, or the nation makes a decision about the length of that person's life. I can understand that. My point is, we need to involve the person as much as possible in such a decision. The person in that altered state of consciousness may be experiencing something very different from what he or she thought would be experienced—and it may be different than anticipated.

For example, I think of an elderly Swiss professor whom Amy and I worked with some years ago in Zurich. He had had a stroke that had left him badly brain damaged. Part of the family wanted to withdraw the life support and the other part of the family knew about our work and called us in. They said, "Before we withdraw the life support, we would like you try to communicate with our husband, father, grandfather, and uncle." We said, "Sure, let's see what happens."

Now this was a man who had said ahead of time that if he got into a coma or state of consciousness that was looking vegetative, he should be allowed to die. So that has to be respected. As we opened the door to his room, he opened his eyes straight ahead, moved his head, and looked toward us. Remember, he had had a stroke, and was pretty badly brain damaged, was in a coma. That's always very shocking! He had been sensing us coming somehow. I said, "We're here." And he went, "Uh-mmm." We had expected to see someone looking nearly like a corpse and here was a person clearly communicating within the limitations of his abilities.

We started to work with him. He had an eyebrow movement; this part of his eyebrow would flicker every now and then [Arny moves one of his eyebrows up]. Now the neurological community will say that this eye flickers like that because of an automatic reflex—meaning, the action takes place without conscious intention or awareness and is meaningless. But in this work, we understand the person as more than just a machine and we assume that the signals they are sending with their body are potentially meaningful.

We focused on that flicker in his eyebrow, saying, "If you want to say 'yes', just make a big flicker, and if you want to say nothing and you don't agree with something, just don't do anything at all." We got a couple of responses from him that showed us he could make that flicker by choice. We also used the movements of his mouth. People who have been in strokes frequently yawn or their mouth will move back and forth. Again, the medical perspective contends those movements are reflexes. We have repeatedly found those movements to be a form of communication.

We got to the point when the whole family was crowded around the bed for the Big Question. I said to him, "Professor, if you'd like to go on living, please make the signs that mean 'yes,' and if you don't care to go on living, because that's a big problem for everyone here, don't make any signs at all." Well, he lifted his eyebrow higher and opened his mouth further than he had since he had been sick! He opened his mouth like this [Arny opens his mouth very widely] and shocked everyone. Clearly he was proclaiming, "Yes, I want to live!" All the whole family members began muttering and pondering. "Wow. What? You want to go on living? Why?"

I went through a bunch of questions getting yeses and noes about why he wanted to go on living. At one point, I said to him, "You want to go on living?" He signaled, yes. "You want to go on living because you want to make more money?" I asked. No response. "You want to go on living because you have some unfinished business in life?" No response. "You want to go on living because you're having a good time where you are?" A big yes! "You're having a good time where you are because you're having a good time on holiday at the coast?" Nothing. "You want to go on living because you're having an affair?" Wow, a huge yes! This guy had led a rather conservative life. He was not the type to have affairs, but now was having an affair in his "comatose" state!

To make the story short—this was an all-night adventure—he was having an affair with a woman while hiking in the mountains. This theme frequently emerges: that people are having affairs with spirit-like lovers just before death.

Anyway, there was no question about it. The family was highly embarrassed. "Grandpa is having an affair. Let's let him live. He's having a good time." That doesn't mean, let him live permanently; that means, let him live moment by moment and the next week ask the same questions again. Several weeks later he signaled that his affair was done and now it would be OK to die. Shortly thereafter, he died.

Following People

We never tell people what to do. No one knows what's right for another person. In everyday life I hate it when people tell me what to do, and I feel the same is true of other people. Follow where people are at—their bodies and their souls will tell you what to do.

We don't force people to come back and communicate. We just say, "Follow where you are, and if you'd like to communicate something, you can communicate it. If you don't feel like communicating and need to go in another direction, you just go ahead and do that, too."

Most medical folks are not trained therapeutically to deal with people in altered states of consciousness. In the medical paradigm, if somebody is not able to communicate in an ordinary state of consciousness, there is something wrong. We view these people as simply being in another state of consciousness. But the medical model is that you have to be in either an ordinary state of consciousness or sleeping, otherwise you're not in order.

That's a pathological view of the human being. It's a good view, it's even a wonderful view for some, but it's not the only view. So many medical people would like to learn to go deeper with their patients but they're shy and afraid and have no education in this area.

Feeling Trapped

Many people want to know if comatose people feel trapped in their bodies. What comatose people experience depends on the state of consciousness they are in. For example, people who are comatose following an accident or brain injury—those people whom I have been able to communicate with—do not feel trapped in a body. The man I just described was having an affair with a spirit of some sort, a dream figure of some sort. So he didn't feel like he was trapped anyplace. On the contrary, he was totally free. On the other hand, some comatose people—when they are almost out of the coma, coming back and becoming more and more awake—begin to experience the frustration they are having in their body at that point.

Learning Coma Work

I always say to students who want to learn more about how to work with people in altered states of consciousness that the first step is to make your own assumptions clear. It's essential to know what your assumptions are, because if you assume that altered states are somehow wrong or pathological, or that there's nobody home, you'd probably be better off doing ordinary medical work. The comatose person senses what your assumptions are, and assumptions such as the above inhibit the person.

The next step is to ask yourself how you feel about death. Is it something to fear? Do you think it's OK for a person to die? You're going to die, probably, one of these days. Is that all right with you? How do you feel about it? What do you think happens in death?

I never tell people what I think happens at death. I always ask, "What do you think happens?" I assume that everyone has very individual experiences in the moments surrounding death, so I'm against programs that say there is a bright light at the end of a tunnel. Some people see that, but many may not. The important point is, what are your assumptions?

The next step is to feel comfortable about approaching people who are in an altered state of consciousness. You can practice with your friends, family, and lovers or partners at home. Go close. Put your cheek next to theirs and speak gently in their ear. Follow their rhythm. Let your own altered states direct you. Get close to the person, try to feel where they are at, and meditate with them, so to speak.

I want to share that the goal is not to get the person to come out of the coma. The goal is not to get the person to let go and die. That is not our business. The goal is to follow nature. Humility is the point. Follow what that person's nature is doing, not what you think they should do, not what the family or medical community thinks they should do. Follow nature itself as much as possible by following the body signals of the person.

Obviously, not everyone is meant to work with comatose people. Some therapists get too upset when they see people in altered states. It's not their cup of tea. A lot of people have been trained only to talk to those whom they are trying to help. Most people in our society, I mean industrial societies, have very little awareness at all about communication outside the verbal realm. In contrast, in Tibet or ancient Egypt it was assumed that we are conscious at the moment of death and even after death.

So coma work is not everybody's cup of tea but a lot of people are interested in altered states of consciousness and would love to know more about coma work. There's usually one family member who takes to it naturally—frequently the quietest, shyest person standing in the corner shaking. Say to her or him, "Sweetheart, would you like to come forward and hold your mother's hand and just speak to her quietly and tell her what you feel in the rhythm of her breathing?" Sometimes a child or loved one is enough to bring a person back. It takes a lot of sensitivity and feeling to communicate with people in this state of consciousness.

What the family's doing around a person in a comatose state may not have as big an effect as people have always thought. The person just stays in their coma until one member of the family comes around who is lovingly gentle and in tune with the comatose person.

The Future

What the future holds for this type of work in the medical community is easy to see from the kind of people who come and train with us. People want to know how to communicate with people in altered states of consciousness. Many of the people in the medical community feel impotent and unhappy just standing by and looking at someone in a coma, washing them and taking care of them.

There is very little in medical science that explains much of what we see around comas. So I have had no debates whatsoever about what happens. In fact, there are neurologists in this country and in Europe who are undertaking studies to track the neurological activities that happen during awakenings.

Noxious Stimulation

In the medical community one of the basic methods for testing if someone's in a comatose state is to apply "noxious stimulation"—a pin prick, different kinds of strong smells, some sort of pain or discomfort introduced to the person. It's understandable that they want to do this, to find out the state of the person's coma, but it seems unnecessarily unrelated to where the person is.

Impact on the Death Process and Grief

There is no doubt in my mind that one of the reasons some people insist that their relatives go on living forever is because they can't communicate with them so they have no way of knowing their wishes. If they knew where the person was at in his or her inner process, they'd be able to say, "Oh, Grandpa is having an affair," or "Grandpa doesn't want to live anymore." Such specific information makes whatever follows—be it the person's death or awakening—more comprehensible. And, I'd say that eighty percent of grieving comes about because people have not been able to communicate with their loved ones in these altered states. It's the lack of communicating that is so painful.

But if you've ever once communicated with someone you've loved who is dying and in an altered state, and heard the depth of experience that she or he is having, it's easier to let go. Afterwards, the amount of grief you experience is eased, though it's always horrible, there's always a terrible sense of loss.

Some people in comas want to communicate with their family and tell them to relax. One person communicated from her coma that she was sorry her coma was going on so long and that her family should go back home and begin life again. She conveyed that she was busy and should be left alone.

But the vast majority do not feel the pain of the family, and family members need to know that their Mama and Papa or Brother or Sister may not be in the same state of consciousness as they were before. So it's not the time necessarily to work out all your unsolved problems with them. Don't go and battle with your father or your mother because you didn't battle during ordinary life. Mama and Papa may not be where they used to be.

What to Remember

When you allow yourself to learn from the death process, you have a much more lighthearted attitude about life. You feel relieved—you don't have to worry about it anymore. The worst thing about death and dying is that you haven't had much experience with it until you get into it yourself. So, learn from those who are dying by communicating with them.

If you want to remember one thing when you go to the hospital and visit somebody, remember that life is an incredible, mysterious experience which you have the great chance of discovering more about with that marvelous teacher who is lying there in bed.

Chapter 16

Nisha Zenoff

I visited with and interviewed Nisha Zenoff in April 1995. Nisha is a friend of ours, a process-oriented therapist and dance-movement therapist, whose mother had died of cancer in 1994.

Nisha was with her mother during her last two months of life, accompanying her through the shock of the diagnosis of cancer, preparation for death, and finally her comatose state just before dying. Arny and I were fortunate to be in contact with Nisha by telephone through much of this process.

Nisha hoped that her experiences and subsequent thoughts about coma work could be of value to others. The kind of communication Nisha had with her mother was an exception to the distance and loneliness many people feel when their loved ones are in strongly altered states as a result of comatose and near-death conditions.

I just had to include this interview with Nisha because she shows, in such a touching manner, how relating to a loved one near death gives us something eternal, something beyond death.

Nisha: Mother was diagnosed with cancer on July 26, and that's when she called me. She said they had found congestion in her lungs, and I thought it sounded very bad. She died on September 21, so it was a little less than two months.

At the age of eighty-one mother still appeared to be full of life, beautiful, strong, and healthy. At seventy-eight, she had taken up golf again and was playing three times a week. When visiting me, she would prune my cacti outside for hours and then express bewilderment that she was tired when she stopped.

When I received the call from her two weeks after her visit, I thought to myself, "This is a call I've been anticipating with dread all my life, the day I would hear that my mother is dying." As a young girl I remember feeling that I could never live without my mother. As a fifty-four-year-old woman, I still couldn't bear the thought.

I knew her death was imminent when the doctor said, "Look, it's just a matter of time. Make sure she lives every day. The only thing we can do is ease the pain. She has the worst kind of advanced cancer."

Arny's suggestion was a surprise. He said, "When your mother's waiting for the diagnosis, don't let her just wait and guess. Tell her that people who have that kind of cancer don't live a long time and she should live every day as if it were her last. Some people die from the shock of waiting for the diagnosis." That was very helpful.

Amy: In what way?

Nisha: It helped me to talk with her directly about her life and her death, which helped her be open and realistic. It helped me to start talking with her about dying and cancer. She didn't want anybody else to know that she had cancer. At first, she called it "my secret," then it became the "C-word" and finally, after a week or two, she was able to call it cancer.

One night, while I was sleeping in her apartment, she suddenly sat up in bed and let out a terrified yell, "Oh, my God, am I dying? Am I dying?" We made the decision that she would stay at home, surrounded by her family, rather than go to the hospital. My brother and I made the decision to call hospice. I phoned them. That was a difficult one, a real acknowledgment that her death was imminent. Six weeks later, she was in a semi-coma.

Amy: What do you mean by a semi-coma? Can you describe it for us?

Nisha: She still whispered and spoke occasionally but her eyes were closed—they never opened again, and she never got out of bed again. Oh, she did actually, with help to get on the potty, but she was in a coma. It was like a deep sleep. She wasn't easily awakened.

Amy: Was she still speaking at this point?

Nisha: Barely. She would whisper slowly and softly. The first morning after she slipped into what seemed to be a coma, her voice was like, "Whaa, waa." She was not on drugs, though they did put her temporarily on morphine later. She said, "How, do you... suppose you... go... about... this? Do you go poof? Or you just go to sleep in the night?" She was speaking slowly and in a muffled tone.

When she asked that question I thought, Oh, my! She's really asking how to die. And I thought, I don't know. I was so shocked to hear her speak, because she hadn't spoken for twenty-four hours and she seemed so deep inside herself. I left the room and meditated and prayed. It took me a couple hours to respond.

I said, "Mom, the important thing is for you to trust and love your inner experience. It doesn't matter if you go poof, or if you just go to sleep in the night. What matters is that you truly, absolutely believe in your experiences." Just like what we had been practicing in our coma classes! I added, "Just love your experience and appreciate it and you'll know the right way."

Amy: Was she making any movements at that time?

Nisha: She made both subtle and surprising movements. One of her lifelong characteristic movements when sleeping was to put her hand over her head, like this, over her forehead. She continued to do it until the day before she died. Sometimes, she couldn't get her arm up there. It would go only this far—halfway to her forehead—and then a little farther. But you could see that movement was happening until the end.

Amy: Did you realize that movement was expressing something important?

Nisha: Yes, with a little help! One night, you and Arny called and said, "What are you doing?" I didn't know what I was doing—I was in such a state. You both said "Do you want to go work with your mother?" and I said, "Absolutely."

So I went into her room. Every now and then, I'd put her on the portable toilet, but she didn't open her eyes. She was quite thin and looked like a younger version of herself. She got more and more beautiful! She no longer looked like eighty years old. The years and wrinkles were melting away.

That night she was just sitting there. Sometimes she would move her arm, and I would gently and slowly pick up her wrist with my thumb and index fingers and wait and watch and assist her to do whatever she was trying to do. Arny said, "There's an experience in there that she is trying to have."

After this experience working with her, while you and Arny were on the phone, I followed her movements in her arms and legs; she moved as if she were flying! Both her arms reached up to the sky, and both her legs moved effortlessly as if she were a bird. At one point she said, "Ducks on the pond." I said, "Really, how many?" She said, "Hundreds and hundreds of ducks, how beautiful!" I wondered if she were looking out, in fantasy, at the ocean bay where I live. She loved the bay. She was flying. She exclaimed,

"Ooohhhhh," ecstatically. I thought the hospice nurse was going to faint!

Amy: You helped her follow and complete her movements?

Nisha: Yes, by following and encouraging them and helping them unfold. She would continue and then stop for a while, then resume. She began moving with her legs and her whole body, and she looked as if she were totally in flight! She was definitely going through something.

For days before, lying in bed, her brow was scrunched. She looked as though she were really concentrating and working hard on her thoughts and experiences inside. But after that movement process, her face totally changed. The change was dramatic. Her face looked at peace and the expression remained. I don't know what her experience was, but it appeared important for her.

Amy: How did the hospice nurse respond?

Nisha: She said she had never seen anything like it. It totally changed her approach from believing she had to fight against the experience and hold her down and not let it come out.

Amy: What do you mean, not let it come out?

Nisha: She was always adjusting Mother, trying to make her more comfortable—what she assumed constituted comfort—rather than encouraging the movement to come forth.

Amy: You mean, she would try to put your mother's arms back down?

Nisha: Exactly. Or she'd put a pillow under her arm. She was always very sweet and loving, but her well-meaning attempts to adjust my mother's body did not follow her movement language.

I could see that encouraging Mother to do what she was doing and using blank access seemed to free her. This approach was very unknown to the nurse. For the human being in an ordinary state of consciousness, this kind of un–self-conscious movement doesn't exist.

But I could see that she breathed more deeply—"huuuh, huuuhhh"—and I followed her lead in her way; it was shifting out of my reality and being in her world. That was the main adjustment.

Amy: That's the big change for most of us.

Nisha: When other family members would see her in bed, they would say, "Oh, my God, she looks awful." And I'd think, what are they talking about? They would be upset because she wouldn't meet them where they were. She didn't talk to them in their language. She didn't greet them with her usual smile and direct eye contact.

I tried to coach them. At one point, I heard my brother say to a relative, "Well, you can visit, but you know, Mom can't talk to you." I was furious! I knew we were continuing to communicate. It didn't occur to me that we weren't! We communicated until she took her last breath! Even when she no longer used words, she was responding and leading the way with her breath, sounds, and her movements!

Amy: Could any of your relatives understand that?

Nisha: Well, my brother really came through. In fact, he sang to her. He sat there and sang love songs to her and held her hand. It just gives me shivers to think about. My daughter (26) and son (28) held her, kissed her, and whispered into her ears, and watched her closely and responded to her reactions.

When the oncologist came to visit, he touched her hand, but barely! And he spoke to her from the foot of the bed. There was a great distance between Mom and him—worlds of distance. And he is considered to be one of the most experienced oncologists around.

I was deeply disappointed that "the experts" did not know how to communicate with her during those final days—her dying days. It was shocking to me, actually. And that is where the loneliness came.

Amy: For you?

Nisha: Yes, for me. Occasionally a friend would visit who knew my mother, and the two of us would be together with her, following her lead. You could see the color change in her face: her face relaxed more and her breathing deepened. I imagine that she felt met or understood or helped.

But then other people would come to visit, expecting her to be in their reality—to greet them with a smile—or pay attention to them as usual. And since she couldn't—or didn't—do those expected things, they assumed she wasn't there.

Amy: Did you feel lonely because you were doing something nobody else understood?

Nisha: Yes. Few understood. I felt excited, though. I couldn't believe some of the things my mother would say and do with her breath and her eyes. She was fully there, even though she was in a coma.

Amy: You are articulating the difference in communication that occurs in different forms of reality so well. Are there any other details that were important to you?

Nisha: Yes, I learned firsthand about spatial proximity. Literally, I would put my lips on her cheeks and on her ear and near her lips and just move them so that she could feel them. Similar to how I would cuddle a baby. Of course, I loved her and this was easy. And then her eyes would move and her breathing would deepen. You could see it. Her skin color would change.

Amy: Yes, someone in my class once said that you know how to do this work if you have held a baby.

Nisha: That's exactly right, Amy. Just like with a baby! She is my mother—but she's not. That's the thing. She transformed from being my mother into someone who's eternal—the eternal.

In ordinary life, I would be too shy to touch my mother like that. In this culture such intimate touch is taboo—it might be labeled sexual or strange or too intimate. And, yet, it didn't matter at that point. I was holding her and caressing her. It was so natural.

Amy: Some people wonder how to be certain that the comatose person would like that kind of contact. What do you think from your experience?

Nisha: Well, I think it's a good question. I followed my feelings. And it is not right for everyone. Touch and physical intimacy are culturally determined. It is an individual matter. Actually that's one reason it helps to practice coma work before you actually need to use it—you can discover where your edges to intimacy and contact are and have opportunities to work with them. You need to follow what you are comfortable with.

Amy: Close contact and intimacy can be a very scary thing for many of us. Can you say more about your experience of this kind of touch?

Nisha: It's about feeling and feedback. The body gives feedback through temperature, movement, the breath. If the person tightens up, you can feel it—the skin subtly pulls away or contracts. It's a sensual, textural sensation you learn to receive—whether the body tightens and pulls or loosens and melts. I always had the feeling my mom was melting.

Some babies, from the beginning, move against you, while others melt into your arms. It was the same thing with my mother. I could tell when I would touch her in a way that was right for her, through her skin. The experience is subtle and not easily described with words. It's an important question, though. My comfort level with her was made far easier by the fact that we had always been comfortable with physical closeness and affection. I grew up being comfortable with my mother.

Amy: That's really helpful.

Nisha: I want to mention another experience. She wasn't eating then, so her mouth got dry. I was no longer brushing her teeth and her teeth got brown. We were wiping her mouth with a cotton swab. That's where she began to change a lot, around the mouth. Her mouth hardly moved anymore.

Amy: So she wasn't making sounds?

Nisha: She would make little sucking motions. At one point Arny suggested I dip one finger in sugar water and then in salt water and alternately put it next to her lips to see if she would suck on it. She responded to the salt water. She bit the tip of my finger really strongly and sucked on it! It was a strong bite. I liked feeling her strong energy.

Amy: Did you have a feeling for where you were going or what your hope was in the way you interacted with your mother?

Nisha: Yes, I was clear that my desire was to make contact with her and assist her. I kept thinking, whatever is happening for her—even if it's strange and I don't understand it—is a natural process. It's her body's way of moving through this. I was trying to honor the unknown, because it was truly unknown. It wasn't medically prescribed or medically assisted.

Amy: Did she seem to be in pain?

Nisha: I asked her if she was in pain. She communicated that she was in pain through big sounds and head nods some of the time, and that's when we started giving her morphine—but she didn't take much morphine. Then Arny recommended that we try cutting back on the morphine, and that's when she became more active and alive. She did not appear to have increased pain, and she seemed to be exploring and completing inner experiences.

Amy: How did you notice that?

Nisha: She was less dreamy and moving around more. Her body made movements that seemed to appear out of nowhere. The absence of morphine took her out of her drugged state, and the pain did not recur. Her facial expression was relaxed and peaceful.

When she died she wasn't on morphine. We stopped it several days before. The nurses couldn't believe it. At first, they didn't want to reduce the morphine, but I said, "This is really important and I want to do it. If she looks like she's in pain, we'll increase it."

Amy: How did the nurses feel about that?

Nisha: They were amazed. Things shifted for them after the experience when Mom appeared to fly. Of course to me and the nurse, my mother was sitting on the pot. But not for my mother! The pot no longer had significance. Isn't that fabulous? She was flying with ducks—at least, that's how it seemed. She looked relaxed and free.

Only right near the end did we hear the "death rattle" in her breathing, but not much. There wasn't much phlegm. The doctor came in and said he had never seen anyone her age so healthy, except for the cancer. She was so healthy. Isn't that incredible? That's how it should be. Giving the body the permission to express its natural self.

At one point the nurse said we might have to give her oxygen, but we didn't. Her breathing was like regular breathing. It was mostly like this, "HHHaahhhh, uhhhh..." [Nisha breathes rather normally but with a very slight strain in each breath]. It didn't get much worse than that. It didn't get much more strained.

Amy: It's so painful when someone dies, but the way you describe this experience, it was also beautiful somehow.

Nisha: It's beautiful to know that death is as natural as birth. It makes me less afraid of my own death. It is the most natural experience. It is such a teaching... to know that the breath just quietly stops.

Amy: Were you there when she died?

Nisha: The nurse called me. She said, "Nisha, come quickly, I think your mother just died." I was in the next room and I walked into her room. Her mouth was slightly open, her eyes were closed, her head was turned to the side, and it was as if she just exhaled, "hhaaa." So that was it. I walked in there, literally, just after she took her last breath. Her body was still warm and I just kept touching her, following and feeling the spirit go out of the physical body and the coolness come.

She had advanced stage-four cancer when it was discovered. She suffered when she went through radiation. She suffered almost two months with diagnosis and prognosis and then with the pain she felt initially. But the death itself was so sacred... so sacred and effortless. She did not suffer. You could see in her expression she no longer had fear. She finally welcomed it. At the end she welcomed death and wasn't afraid.

Amy: Oh, that's amazing. Thanks for sharing those experiences, Nisha. Was there anything else that stood out to you that you feel is important for others to know?

Nisha: One of the most important things—and this is why the coma training is so important—is that the way of interacting becomes second nature. I truly believe what I said to my mother: "Believe in your experience, Mother, it's OK.

What needs to happen is already happening in you. Please trust it." I could say it... it just makes me cry... I could honestly say it because I believe it.

Amy: That's perhaps the deepest love you can give someone.

Nisha: Yes. I could say, "Truly, Mother, please believe that your experience is exactly what you need in the moment." And that helped her, I think, more than anything, because it helped her not be afraid. When she said her senses were changing, I could say, "That's right, and you don't need regular food anymore, your food comes from a different place, a spiritual nourishment." And when she was making sounds, I amplified her sounds to accompany her.

Amy: Did you have the feeling that she could hear you all the time?

Nisha: Absolutely! I never doubted for a second that she was hearing me. The muscles in her face reacted. There was so much life. This is the point. When I heard my brother say that Mother wasn't talking anymore, I was upset. But then I realized that, to him, communicating is when you sit up and look at each other in the eye, and you talk in a related way, like we do in "normal" conversation.

But for me, because of training in coma work, that no longer was the guideline. Communication was the blinking of her eyes or the rolling of the eyeballs under the lids when they were closed. Or it was the slight movement in the muscles in her jaw. It was the movement of her breath changing from shallow to deep, or deep to shallow. It was the external movements of the periphery of her body.

It was like talking in another language without realizing that I was communicating in another language. Like using Spanish or dreaming in Spanish without realizing I had shifted from English.

Amy: Right, a whole other language.

Nisha: The language comes through the body. It doesn't only come through verbal communication. And to speak the language of the body isn't a matter of just watching it but feeling it, too.

Amy: Nisha, if you were to advise people about this work, is there a particular message you'd want people to know?

Nisha: A couple of things. One is about entering the other person's experience, not standing outside it and looking at it. You have to get in there with them, so that the distance between the realities is less. Before my mother went into a coma she told me a dream. She and I were in a canoe just sailing along. I took that to mean I had to get in there with her—and just sail along together.

Coma work requires practice—it's building a skill and an endurance of sorts. I think it's like riding a bicycle. You get on and you ride and practice, and then one day, if you want to ride in a triathlon, the muscles and endurance are built up. The skill is there. It's like an athletic skill or playing scales on the piano. Then when you are in a crisis, or when you are racing against time and death is near, you are ready. I think the more we sit with each other in classes and clinics, the more we practice with each other, the more the work becomes second nature.

However, I also know that many people who are in a crisis can learn basic skills by receiving coaching from someone who is experienced in coma work. Sometimes this can even be done over the telephone—as you well know.

Whether you put your finger inside somebody's lips and touch their teeth or put your face next to their face or feel their breathing, it's just natural. It helps to work on our own edges to this type of physical closeness.

Amy: It seems foolish that we don't learn this kind of communication from the beginning—though, of course, we all communicate like this as children.

Nisha: We do it as children but then unlearn it and are taught in this culture not to value it. What does it mean to believe in your own experience? I knew my mother was dying, I knew there was an outcome. What she was going through was leading her to that outcome. There's something about believing in personal experience, knowing it's purposeful.

What is the purpose of it? The hospice nurse said, "Why do you want to do this? Don't disturb her. She just needs to be peaceful and comfortable." And I'd think, "Why not disturb her?" What I was doing may have looked like a disturbance, but it seemed helpful to her.

Amy: What do you think about that now?

Nisha: What I saw—when her brows were furrowed—looked like she was working very intently on something internally that wasn't getting resolved. When I assisted and followed her physically and supported her movement and her experiences, something in her appearance shifted, something released and the result was noticeably a more peaceful state. It's about helping someone die congruently!

Amy: Without conflict, you mean?

Nisha: That's it. That's what it was. Dying congruently means dying without unfinished business. It's not only the survivors who have unfinished business; it appears that the person who is trying to die or not trying to die is working internally on her stuff, too.

Amy, there is that which doesn't die—even in the midst of the physical body dying (perhaps a topic for another book). And that "something"— that eternal something that doesn't die, that is always there—was so strong. I felt it so strongly during this time with my mom. Her death was as natural as natural childbirth. No struggle, no tubes—a natural passing of the physical body. What an honor to bear witness to this moment of dying—the separating of what is eternal from that which is not.

What a gift to witness such a beautiful and gentle passing. To know that death is natural and can be gentle and easy. What a teaching. I am so grateful.

Coma work bridges ordinary reality with the deepest altered state of consciousness—coma. By shifting modes of communication through the use of sound, movement, touch, and rhythm, you adapt to the comatose person's "language." There, in that seemingly unreachable state, you discover the dreams, fantasies, inner experiences, and desires of your loved ones, friends, and patients. You join comatose people at a deep, intimate level and can ask them important questions.

By the time you read this, you will have gone through many experiences with a comatose person, or with other learners, and you will have had many of your own personal journeys. Whether you are a helping professional, therapist, family member, or friend, it is time to take a breath, to re-feel what you have experienced, and to consider your next steps.

Coma work awakens all of us to the often unnoticed depths of human experience. It brings each of us to the brink of the most elemental questions about life, about death, and about the meaning of human existence. Perhaps contact with comatose people will remind us of the vastness of our own experience and will propel us to draw closer to the profound inner stream that guides our lives. As we enter this current, we live more fully, throughout the entirety of life.

Altered state of consciousness—Any state of consciousness that is different from the state we ordinarily identify with. Typical altered states of consciousness include drowsiness, intense anger, or falling in love. Altered states can happen willfully, for example, through the use of drugs or high levels of exercise, or involuntarily, such as through the onset of coma. Coma is the deepest altered state of consciousness.

Amplification—The intensification or expansion and deepening of experiences.

Binary communication—A nonverbal method of asking questions that can be answered with a simple yes or no.

Blank access—A technique that uses noninterpretive or "blank" words, sounds, and movements to help amplify experiences.

Brain death—Clinically and legally viewed today as the irreversible loss of brainstem function.

Brain injury—Mechanical injury to the brain attributable to traumatic or non-traumatic sources. Traumatic sources include accidents, strokes, or blood hemorrhages. Non-traumatic sources include brain tumors, hypoxia, drug overdose, and alcoholism.

Cerebrospinal fluid—A clear fluid that surrounds and protects the brain and spinal cord.

Channels—Sensory-oriented pathways or modes through which we perceive. Among the most common channels are kinesthetic (movement), auditory, proprioceptive (feeling), and visual channels.

Coma—In the medical context, a prolonged state of unresponsiveness much like sleep in which the person does not react to outer stimuli or to her inner needs. The comatose state may be due to metabolic, structural, or psychogenic factors, or a combination of these. From a process-oriented viewpoint, coma is an extreme altered state of consciousness in which the person is not relating to ordinary reality, yet is going through potentially meaningful inner experiences and can be related to through special communication methods.

In this manual, the term *coma* is used broadly to refer to a spectrum of altered states from the deepest form of coma to a persistent vegetative state, and to the various stages in which the person emerges into degrees of wakefulness and recovery. Some of these are defined medically by such terms as clouding of consciousness, delirium, stupor, locked-in syndrome, and the minimally responsive state.

Congruence—When the body, or parts of the body, function as a unified system.

Consciousness—From a medical standpoint (and in relationship to coma) the awareness of self and environment. In this context, coma is the opposite condition—that of unconsciousness—in which there is no awareness of oneself or the environment, even when stimulated externally. In a process-oriented model the degree of consciousness is assessed by discovering the comatose person's potential for inner awareness and perception, as well as responses to outer communication that are related to the comatose person's altered state of consciousness.

Consensus reality—The definitions of reality (and therefore of all communication methods) that are implicitly agreed upon by a given culture.

CT scan—Computerized tomography scan. A test that uses a combination of computer and x-ray technology to reveal physical abnormalities by means of high-quality, cross-sectional views of body tissues.

Decerebrate posturing—Characteristic positioning of the hands and fingers in which the arms are extended outward rigidly and turned away from the center of the body as a result of injury to particular motor areas of the brain.

Decorticate posturing—Characteristic positioning of the hands and fingers in which they are rigidly bent in and upward toward the chest as a result of injury to particular motor areas of the brain.

Deep bodywork—The use of the hands in a loving way to elicit profound body experiences.

Diffuse brain injury—Brain injury that affects many areas of the brain, typically caused by a buildup of poisonous substances that intoxicate brain tissues or by prolonged hypoxia.

Double-state ethics—An ethical standpoint that incorporates the responses of the person before he went into a coma, as well as responses while in the coma, about life-and-death issues.

Edge—The boundary to our known identity. On one side of the edge is the way we normally identify ourselves; on the other side are all the numinous, mysterious, and unknown aspects of our experiences and potentials.

EEG—Electroencephalogram. A test that measures the electrical activity within the brain, revealing whether the person is alert, awake, or asleep.

Feedback—In coma, feedback means communication responses from the comatose person to your communications through the use of movements, sounds, changes in breathing, coloration changes in the skin, and so forth.

Fundamental body communication—The most elemental ways in which we communicate through the use of the eyes, mouth, breath, sounds, lips, hands, and movements of the limbs.

Glasgow Coma Scale—A scale that measures the level of consciousness in people who have sustained brain injuries.

Hospice—An approach to terminal care of the dying person that stresses comfort, as well as quality-of-life issues and the desires of the patient and family. It is a palliative rather than a cure-based approach.

Hypoxia—Insufficient amount of oxygen in the blood and lungs, which can lead to brain injury.

Living will—A document in which a person in her ordinary state of consciousness states what care she would like if death is imminent and life-sustaining procedures would only delay the moment of death. This is one of a number of documents called "advance directives."

Localized brain injury—Brain trauma occurring at a particular area of the brain and causing specific defects in the function of the brain; depending on the place of injury, defects may include loss of coordination, difficulty with speech, or paralysis.

Metabolic coma—Coma attributable to an alteration in blood chemistry, which results in a general reduction of the body's ability to function normally and which has not developed to the point of structural damage to the brain. The metabolic coma often occurs near death; causes include severe insulin imbalances, situations near death when the sodium/potassium balance is disrupted, and toxins.

Metaskills—The feeling attitudes that accompany technical skills. The metaskills of coma work include love, openness, compassion, patience, a beginner's mind, and sentient awareness.

Minimal cues—Minute signals, such as slight movements of the mouth, eyebrows, and fingers and slight alterations of the breath.

Morphine—A synthetic narcotic used to induce sleep and relieve pain.

MRI—Magnetic resonance imaging. A test that reveals physical abnormalities by means of high-quality, cross-sectional views of body tissues without the use of x-rays or other forms of irradiation.

Pacing the breath—Joining the comatose person's breathing rate by adjusting your verbal and physical interventions to this rhythm.

Palliative care—Care that emphasizes increasing the quality of a person's life and the management of pain.

Persistent vegetative state—A state in which the person appears awake but is seemingly unresponsive and the sleep/wake cycle returns. This is sometimes called *akinetic mutism, coma vigil,* or *appalic syndrome.* Some comatose individuals enter this state after emerging from the deepest form of coma.

Physical therapy—Physical treatment of injuries and disorders by means of such methods as massage, exercise, cold and hot treatments, or electrical current, which are used to guard against atrophy, reduce joint stiffness, strengthen muscles, and retrain muscles and joints.

Primary process—All aspects of experience that connect with our ordinary identity.

Process—The flow of signals through various sensory-oriented channels.

Process-oriented approach—An approach based on following the natural process, or flow of signals, of an individual, in contrast to a predetermined program.

Psychogenic coma—Coma that is linked to psychological factors such as mania or depression. Some psychological states, such as catatonia, mimic coma.

Rancho Los Amigos Coma Scale of Cognitive Functioning—A scale for charting stages of recovery in head-injured individuals.

Sculpting—A method of bodywork in which the hands are used like those of a sensitive potter to access inner body experiences.

Secondary process—All aspects of our experience that we perceive as lying outside our ordinary identity.

Sensitive communication—Communication that is adapted to the altered state of the comatose person and adjusts to his feedback.

Sensory-oriented—Related to the sensory experiences such as movement, feeling, hearing, and seeing.

Sentient awareness—The awareness of sentient experience through the use of intuition, feeling, or sensitive touch, or a combination of these.

Sentient experience—Preverbal, subtle feelings and tendencies.

Signals—Bits of information, such as grimaces, changes of skin color, movements, sounds, shallow or deep breaths, and twitches.

Structural coma—A coma attributable to mechanical damage to the brain resulting from traumatic or non-traumatic sources.

Thanatos ethics—Ethical viewpoints about death.

Unfolding—Deepening an experience so that it begins to spontaneously express or generate itself and flow naturally.

Ventilator—A machine that takes over breathing, thereby sustaining life. Also called a life-support machine.

Books, Articles, and Publications

Aitken Neuroscience Institute. "Guidelines for the Management of Severe Head Injury." New York: The Institute, 1995.

American Congress of Rehabilitation Medicine. "Recommendations for Use of Uniform Nomenclature Pertinent to Patients with Severe Alterations in Consciousness." *Archives of Physical Medicine and Rehabilitation* 76, no. 2 (February 1995): 205–9.

Andrews, Keith. "Managing the Persistent Vegetative State." *British Medical Journal* 305, no. 6852 (August 1992): 486–7.

Andrews, Keith, L. Murphy, R. Munday, and C. Littlewood. "Misdiagnosis of the Vegetative State: Retrospective Study in a Rehabilitation Unit." *British Medical Journal*, Vol. 313, no. 7048, (July 1996): 13–16.

Bauby, Jean-Dominique. *The Diving Bell and the Butterfly.* New York: Alfred A. Knopf, 1997.

Bennet, Donald R. *Atlas of Electroencephalography in Coma and Cerebral Death: EEG at the Bedside or in the Intensive Care Unit.* New York: Raven Press, 1976.

Beresford, Larry. *The Hospice Handbook: A Complete Guide.* Foreword by Elisabeth Kubler-Ross. Boston: Little, Brown, 1993.

Black, Henry Campbell. *Black's Law Dictionary.* 6th ed. St. Paul, MN: West Publishing Co., 1990.

Blakely, Mary Kay. *Wake Me When It's Over.* New York: Times Books, 1990.

Bobath, Berta. *Abnormal Postural Reflex Activity Caused by Brain Lesions.* Oxford: Butterworth-Heinemann, 1991.

The Book of the Dead. With a New Introduction by David Lorimer. New York: Penguin Books, 1989.

Brain Injury Association, Inc. "Basic Questions About Brain Injury and Disability." Washington, D.C.: The Association.

Brannon, Joyce, D.A. Coyne, and B. McLeroy. *You Are Not Alone: A Handbook for Hospice Caregiving.* Ann Arbor, MI: Hospice of Washtenaw, 1992.

Byrne, John, J., ed. "The Management of Shock and Unconsciousness." *The Surgical Clinics of North America* 48, no. 2 (April 1968): 245-466.

Callanan, Maggie and Patricia Kelley. *Final Gifts: Understanding the Special Awareness, Needs and Communication of the Dying.* New York: Bantam Books, 1992.

Castenada, Carlos. *Journey to Ixtlan: The Lessons of Don Juan.* Hammondsworth, Middlesex, England: Penguin, 1972.

Choi, Sung C., R.K. Narayan, R.L. Anderson, J.D. Ward. "Enhanced Specificity of Prognosis in Severe Head Injury." *Journal of Neurosurgery* 69 (September 1988): 381–5.

Chuang, S. "Neuroradiological Findings in the Comatose Child." In *Coma: Psychopathology, Diagnosis and Management.* Edited by L. P. Ivan and Derek A. Bruce. Springfield, Ill: Charles C. Thomas, 1982.

Clayman, Charles B., ed. *The American Medical Association Encyclopedia of Medicine.* New York: Random House, 1989.

"Coma: Its Treatment and Consequences." Washington, D.C. Brain Injury Association, Inc., Pamphlet CEM: 83-004.

The Diagram Group. *The Brain: A User's Manual.* New York: Perigee Books, 1982.

Doman, Glenn, R. Wilkinson, M. Dimancescu, R. Pelligra. "The Effect of Intense Multi-sensory Stimulation on Coma Arousal and Recovery." *Neurophyschological Rehabilitation,* 3, no. 2 (1993): 203-212.

Duda, Deborah. *Coming Home: A Guide to Home Care for the Terminally Ill.* Santa Fe, N.M.: John Muir Publications, 1984.

Eliade, Mircea. *Shamanism: Archaic Techniques of Ecstasy.* Bollingen Series 76. Princeton, N.J.: Princeton University Press, 1964.

Egyptian Book of the Dead. Translated and transliterated by E.A. Wallis Budge. New York: Dover, 1967.

Evans-Wentz, W.Y., ed. *The Tibetan Book of the Dead.* London: Oxford University Press, 1960.

Fahrlaender, H. "Medizinische, Rechtliche und Ethische Probleme bei Permanentem Vegetativem Zustand." *Medizinische Wochenschrift,* 126 (1996): 1187–95.

Fazekas, Joseph F., and Ralph W. Alman. *Coma: Biochemistry, Physiology and Therapeutic Principles.* American Lectures in Chemistry Series, Publication 5-7. Springfield, Ill.: Charles C. Thomas, 1962.

Frankowski, Ralph R., John F. Annegers, and Steven Whitman. "Epidemiological and Descriptive Studies. Part I. The Descriptive Epidemiology of Head Trauma in the United States." In *Central Nervous System Trauma Status Report.* Edited by D. P. Becker and J. Povlishock. Bethesda, MD: National Institute of Neurological and Communicative Disorders and Stroke, 1985.

Freeman, E.A., ed. *The Catastrophe of Coma: A Way Back.* Dobbs Ferry, N.Y.: Sheridan Medical Books, 1987.

Friend, Tim. "Seeking Clear-headed Conversation About Coma." *USA Today,* February 26, 1996.

Garrison, Jayne. "Rushing Heaven's Door." *Health Magazine,* May/June 1997, 123–9.

Giacino, Joseph T., and Nathan D. Zasler. "Outcome After Severe Traumatic Brain Injury: Coma, the Vegetative State, and the Minimally Responsive State." *Journal of Head Trauma Rehabilitation* 10, no. 1 (February 1995): 40–56.

Gilfix, Michael, Myra Gerson Gilfix, and Kathleen S. Sinatra. "The Persistent Vegetative State." *Journal of Head Trauma Rehabilitation* 1, no. 1 (March 1986): 63–71.

Gladwell, Malcolm. "Conquering the Coma." *The New Yorker,* July 8, 1996, 34-40.

Goodman, Ellen. "Choosing Life or Death for the Future Self." *International Herald Tribune,* March 8, 1996.

Gow, Christina M., and J. Ivan Williams. "Nurses' Attitudes Toward Death and Dying: A Causal Interpretation." *Social Science and Medicine,* 11 (February 1977): 191–8.

"Guidelines on the Termination of Life-Sustaining Treatment and the Care of the Dying: A Report by the Hastings Center." Bloomington, Ind.: Indiana University Press, 1987.

Hagen, Chris, Danese Malkmus, and Patricia Durham. "Rancho Los Amigos Levels of Cognitive Functioning." Downey, CA: Rancho Los Amigos Medical Center, 1972.

Halifax, Joan. *Shaman: The Wounded Healer.* London: Thames and Hudson, 1982.

Harner, Michael. *The Way of the Shaman.* New York: Bantam Books, 1980.

Hern, Adele. *Vancouver Island Head Injury Society Newsletter,* Fall 1991.

Humphry, Derek. *Final Exit: The Practicalities of Self-Deliverance and Assisted Suicide for the Dying.* Secausus, N.J.: Hemlock Society, 1991.

Ivan, L.P., and E.G. Ventureyra. "Coma and the Evolution of Brain Resuscitation in Coma." In *Coma: Physiopathology, Diagnosis and Management.* Edited by L.P. Ivan and Derek A. Bruce. Springfield, Ill.: Charles C. Thomas, 1982.

Jacobs, Harvey E., Craig A. Muir, and James D. Cine. "Family Reactions to the Persistent Vegetative State." *Journal of Head Trauma Rehabilitation* 1, no. 1 (March 1986): 55–62.

Jennett, Bryan. *Management of Head Injuries*. Philadelphia: F. A. Davis, 1981.

Jonsen, Albert R., Mark Siegler, and William J. Winslade. *Clinical Ethics: A Practical Approach to Ethical Decision in Clinical Medicine*. New York: Macmillan, 1982.

Kearney, Michael. *Mortally Wounded: Stories of Soul Pain, Death and Healing*. Dublin: Marino Books, 1996.

Kolplan, Kenneth I., ed. "Medicolegal Issues: Functional Outcome Evaluation of the Head Injured: Its Effect on Legal Rights." *Journal of Head Trauma and Rehabilitation* 2, no. 3 (September 1987): 93.

Korein, Julius, ed. "Brain Death: Interrelated Medical and Social Issues." *Annals of the New York Academy of Sciences*, 315 (November 1978): 6-18.

Kubler-Ross, Elisabeth. *On Death and Dying*. New York: Macmillan, 1969.

———. *Death: The Final Stage of Growth*. Englewood Cliffs, N.J.: Prentice-Hall, 1975.

Lemley, Brad. "Back from Coma." *New Age Journal*, September/October 1994, 80–3, 150–4.

Leviton, Richard. "Mysteries of the Coma." *East/West Magazine*, September 1990.

Levine, Stephen. *Who Dies? An Investigation Into Conscious Living and Dying*. New York: Doubleday, 1982.

———. *Meetings at the Edge: Dialogues with the Grieving and the Dying, the Healing and the Healed*. Garden City, N.Y.: Anchor Press, 1984.

LeWinn, Edward B. *Coma Arousal*. Garden City, N.Y.: Doubleday, 1985.

Lewis, M.L. and I.C. Colliet. *Medical Surgical Nursing*. St. Louis: Mosby–Year Book, 1992.

Linge, Frederick R. "What Does It Feel Like to Be Brain Damaged?" *Canada's Mental Health* 28, no. 3, (September 1980): 4–7.

Little, Deborah Whiting. *Home Care for the Dying*. Garden City, N.Y.: Doubleday, 1985.

Lundkvist, Artur. *Journeys in Dream and Imagination: The Hallucinatory Memoir of a Poet in a Coma*. New York: Four Walls Eight Windows, 1991.

Menon, D.K. et al. "Cortical Processing in Persistent Vegetative States." *The Lancet*, 352 (July 18, 1998): 200.

Mindell (Kaplan), Amy. "The Hidden Dance: Working With Movement in Process-Oriented Psychology." Thesis. Yellow Springs, Ohio: Antioch University, 1986.

Mindell, Amy. *Metaskills: The Spiritual Art of Therapy*. Tempe, Ariz.: New Falcon Publications, 1995.

Mindell, Amy and Arnold. *Riding the Horse Backwards: Process Work in Theory and Practice*. New York and London: Penguin/Arkana, 1992.

Mindell, Arnold. *A Modern Shaman's Guide to the Universe*. Forthcoming.

———. *City Shadows: Psychological Interventions in Psychiatry*. New York and London: Penguin (Arkana), 1988.

———. *Coma: The Dreambody Near Death*. New York and London: Penguin (Arkana), 1994. Reprint of Coma: Key to Awakening. Boulder, Colo.: Shambhala, 1989.

———. *Dreambody*. Santa Monica, Calif.: Sigo Press, 1982. Reprint, London: Penguin (Arkana) 1988; Portland, Ore.: Lao Tse Press, 1998.

———. *Working With the Dreaming Body*. London: Routledge and Kegan Paul, 1984. Reprint, London and New York: Penguin (Arkana), 1988.

———. *The Mastermind*. Forthcoming.

———. *The Shaman's Body*. San Francisco: HarperCollins, 1993.

———. *Twenty-four Hour Lucid Dreaming*. Forthcoming

Moody, Raymond. *Life After Life*. New York: Bantam Books, 1975.

Multi-Society Task Force on the PVS. "Medical Aspects of PVS: Statement of the Multi-Society Task Force. Part I." *New England Journal of Medicine* 330, no. 21 (May 1994): 1499–508.

———. "Medical Aspects of PVS: Statement of the Multi-Society Task Force." Part II. *New England Journal of Medicine* 330, no. 22 (June 1994): 1572–9.

Neidhardt, J. G. *Black Elk Speaks: Being the Life Story of a Holy Man of the Oglala Sioux.* Lincoln, NB: University of Nebraska Press, 1932.

Nicholson, Shirley, ed. *Shamanism: An Expanded View of Reality.* Wheaton, Ill.: Theosophical Publishing House, 1987.

Osis, Darlis, and Erlendur Haraldsson. *At the Hour of Death.* New York: Avon Books, 1977.

Plum, F. and J.B. Posner. *The Diagnosis of Stupor and Coma.* 3rd ed. Contemporary Neurology Series 19, Philadelphia: FA Davis, 1980.

Prashker, B.A., ed. *The Columbia University College of Physicians and Surgeons Complete Home Medical Guide.* 3rd ed. New York: Crown Publishers, 1995.

President's Commission for the Study of Ethical Problems in Medicine and Biomedical and Behavioral Research. *Defining Death: Medical, Legal and Ethical Issues in the Determination of Death.* Washington, D.C., 1981.

Quinlan, Joseph and Julie. *Karen Ann: The Quinlans Tell Their Story.* Garden City, N.Y.: Doubleday, 1977.

Ring, Kenneth. *Heading Toward Omega: In Search of the Meaning of the Near-Death Experience.* New York: William Morrow, 1984.

Rinpoche, Sogyal. *The Tibetan Book of Living and Dying.* San Francisco: HarperCollins, 1992.

Ross, Kay. "A Comparison of the Medical/Nursing and Process Work Approaches to Coma: A Journey Through the Minefield of Unconsciousness." *Journal of Process Oriented Psychology* 5, no. 2, (Fall/Winter 1993): 23–31.

Slater, Beverly, with Maria Kendricksen and Barbara Zoltan. *Coping With Head Injury.* Thorofare, N.J.: Slack, Inc., 1988.

Stoddard, Sandol. *The Hospice Movement.* New York: Vintage Books, 1978.

Tart, Charles. *Altered States of Consciousness.* New York: Wiley, 1969.

Taylor, Hedley. *The Hospice Movement in Britain: Its Role and Its Future.* London: Centre for Policy on Aging, 1983.

Tomandl, Stan. *Coma Work and Palliative Care: An Introductory Communication Skills Manual for Supporting People Living Near Death.* Victoria, B.C.: White Bear Books, 1991.

Tyson, George W. *Head Injury Management for Providers of Emergency Care.* Baltimore: Williams & Wilkins, 1987.

Vancouver Island Head Injury Society. "Traumatic Head Injury." Victoria, B.C.: The Society, 1991.

Victoria Hospice Society. *Hospice Resource Manual.* Vol. 1, Medical Care of the Dying. Victoria, B.C.: The Society, 1990.

Young, Bryan, Warren Blume, and Abbyann Lynch. "Brain Death and the Persistent Vegetative State: Similarities and Contrasts." *The Canadian Journal of Neurological Sciences* 16, no. 4 (November 1989): 388–93.

Young, George. "Hospice and Health Care." In *Hospice: The Living Idea.* Edited by Cicely Saunders, Dorothy H. Summers, and Neville Teller. London: Edward Arnold, 1981.

Whyte, John, and Mel Bo Glenn. "The Care and Rehabilitation of the Patient in a Persistent Vegetative State." *Journal of Head Trauma Rehabilitation* 1, no. 1 (March 1986): 39–53.

Zaleski, Carol. *Otherworld Journeys: Accounts of Near-Death Experience in Medieval and Modern Times.* New York: Oxford University Press, 1987.

Organizations

Aitken Neuroscience Institute, 523 E. 72nd St., New York, N.Y. 10021.

Brain Injury Association, Inc., 1776 Massachusetts Ave. NW, Suite 100, Washington, DC 20036.

Lao Tse Press, P.O. Box 8898, Portland, Ore. 97207. Publications on process-oriented psychology and process work, including *The Journal of Process Oriented Psychology.*

National Institute of Neurological Disorders and Stroke, Bldg. 31, Rm. 806, 31 Center Dr., MSC 2540, Bethesda, MD 20892.

New Dimensions Radio, P.O. Box 4105, San Francisco, CA 94141.

The Institutes for the Achievement of Human Potential, 8801 Stenton Ave., Philadelphia, PA 19038.

Thinking Allowed Productions, 2560 9th St., Suite 123, Berkeley, CA 94710.

Upledger Institute, 11211 Prosperity Farms Road, Palm Beach Gardens, FL 33410-3487.

Vancouver Island Head Injury Society, 109-1450 Hillside Ave., Victoria, B.C., V8T 2B7, Canada. Publications on traumatic brain injury.

Victoria Hospice Society, 1900 Fort St., Victoria, B.C., V8R 1J8, Canada.

White Bear Books, Box 5575, Station B, Victoria, B.C., V8R 6S4, Canada.

Zen Hospice Project, 273 Page St., San Francisco, CA 94102.

Audiotapes, Videotapes, and Television Programs

"Coma." Program in the *Nova* series. Public Broadcasting Service, October 7, 1997.

"Coma: The Silent Epidemic." The Discovery Channel, November 3, 1997.

"Coma: Work With the Dying." Interview with Arnold Mindell. San Francisco: Thinking Allowed Productions, 1988. Videotape.

Giacino, Joseph T., Douglas I. Katz, Jay Rosenberg, Nathan D. Zasler, and John Whyte. "The Vegetative and Minimally Responsive States: Development of Practical Guidelines." Presented at the 14th Annual National Symposium of the Brain Injury Association. San Diego, CA: Sound of Knowledge, Inc., December 5, 1995. Tape 14A. Audiotape.

———. "Consumer Forum about Practice Guidelines for the Vegetative and Minimally Responsive States." Presented at the 14th Annual National Symposium of the Brain Injury Association. San Diego: CA: Sound of Knowledge, Inc., December 5, 1995. Tape 43. Audiotape.

———. "Primary Care Innovations for Persons With Traumatic Brain Injury." Presented at the 14th Annual National Symposium of the Brain Injury Association. San Diego, CA: Sound of Knowledge, Inc., December 5, 1995. Tape 46. Audiotape.

"Your Body Speaks Its Dreams." Interview with Arnold Mindell. San Francisco: New Dimensions Radio, 1988. Audiotape.

"Waking Up From the Dream." Interview with Amy and Arnold Mindell. San Francisco: New Dimensions Radio, 1989. Audiotape.

Anatomy, Movement, Body Connections, and Bodywork

Calais-Germain, Blandine. *Anatomy of Movement*. Seattle: Eastland Press, 1993.

Kapit, Wynn, and Lawrence M. Elson. *The Anatomy Coloring Book*. 2nd ed. New York: Canfield Press, 1993.

Olsen, Andrea. *Body Stories: A Guide to Experiential Anatomy*. Barrytown, N.Y.: Station Hill Press, 1991.

Raheem, Aminah. *Process Acupressure*. Palm Beach Gardens, FL: Upledger Institute, 1996.

Smith, Fritz. *Inner Bridges: Zero Balancing*. Atlanta: Humanics, New Age, 1986.

Tortora, Gerard J. and Sandra R. Grabowski. *Principles of Anatomy and Physiology*. 7th ed. New York: HarperCollins, 1993.

For information about coma work:

Amy Mindell, Ph.D.
c/o Process Work Center of Portland
2049 NW Hoyt St.
Portland, OR 97209
USA

Index